The Courageous
SELF-LOVE
JOURNEY

Erica Glessing, Editor

Happy Publishing

www.HappyPublishing.net

Table of Contents

Foreword

Dr. Kathleen McNulty, PhD

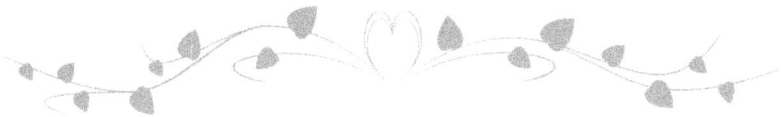

How is it that we don't take very good care of ourselves? How is it that self-love is diminished yet we put others on pedestals? What is Self-Love? Is Self-Love innate or something we learn or both. Can our ability to Self-Love be damaged? Our God self, the spark of the divinity within us is perfect and is Love. It is our human self that can become damaged and disfigured.

Self-reflection aids us in understanding our self needs and promotes self-love. How does self-love develop? From infancy we are vulnerable, small humans. We are dependent on the external world to care for us and meet our basic needs. What if our basic needs go unmet? How does this affect the infant? What blueprint is developing in the infant brain? Emotional coding is being translated onto the neuronal map of the human brain. This in turn has the potential of

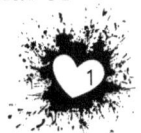

creating skewed perceptions of the outside world, i.e., it is unsafe, no one cares for you, you are not worthy and you are "UNLOVABLE". As human beings we are wired for love. We grow and develop in relationship to "others". We are initially dependent on caretakers to provide basic needs and LOVE for us. A loving, caring relationship between caregiver and infant wires the infant for self-love. The human infant learns and incorporates that he/she is lovable and a healthy program of "self-love" is installed in the human brain, the neuronal bunches if you will. We are wired to self-love and to love others. You ask: "What is possible if early life did not go so well"? The divine created this human organism to heal earlier wounds and developmental insults. There are multiple avenues for healing. One avenue is while in therapeutic relationship with other loving humans who will provide what was missing in early life. These relationships serve as reflections of the "self" so that reparenting can occur and the human brain will develop new neuronal pathways and bundles discarding the old "neglect of self-programs" in favor of self-love. This, in turn, shifts perception in the human brain/mind and the outside world is seen as a safe, trusting and loving. A more balanced perception allows the mind to create adjustments in trust. Intuition develops as yet another avenue to discern who is trust worthy and safe. Self-love develops and is inter-dependent on the collective Love (All of humanity).

Therefore, Love for others and self is paramount in this life. Loving yourself promotes the collective love.

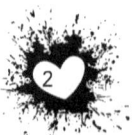

Collective Love promotes the goodness and soul growth of humanity. May this book on Self-Love ignite your soul to assist in further developing your ability to self-love thus adding to the collective soul of humanity here on Earth. Stand in front of a mirror and say: "I love myself. I love you".

Kathleen McNulty, PhD

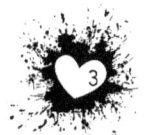

Chapter 1

The Most Valuable Product

Grace Engel

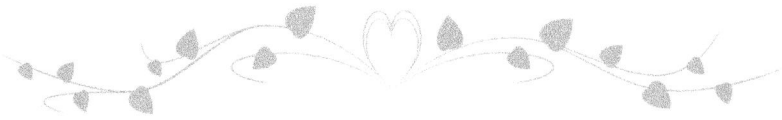

"I've always been the woman of my dreams."
~ Nayyirah Waheed

Self-love is something we're not taught. What we're taught, and what's considered to be the most valuable product, from our first breath, is being good! Be a good child, get good grades, build a good career, be a good employee, start a good family, be a good spouse...

Much of our lives is based on definitions and imposed constructs. We learn to not trust what is true for us.

Constructs —
I should be...
...a lawyer
...a doctor
...a dentist

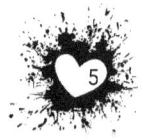

I should never be… me.

These definitions and constructs have taught us to seek validation outside ourselves. We seek to be validated by a career, titles, assets, ultimately eroding the beauty and essence of you.

We are not taught that the most valuable product is you!

If the gift of you has been eroded from birth, it's no wonder self-love has become a dying art.

When someone asks you to be you, you say, "Be who?" Questions arise such as: Who am I? What does it mean to be me? How do I be me without judging myself?

I once read a powerful word:

> "you
> see your face.
> you
> see a flaw.
> how. if you are the only one that has this face?"
> — Nayyirah Waheed

These constructs strip us from receiving, trusting, knowing that inside of you, you have valuable resources that cannot be depleted. Infinite beauty, wisdom, knowledge, truth, wealth, brilliance, creativity — reside within you.

All that is required is for you to walk in your light…

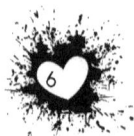

When you start acknowledging that you are a gift, the constructs fall to the wayside. You start to see you, the you that has always been there and never left. You see your beauty; you fall in love with you.

Good, bad, ugly, you embrace all of you. You see beyond the lies perpetuated on you from birth and you no longer need to chase acknowledgement, validation, being liked, fitting in, and being chosen.

You don't need to chase anyone's beauty.
You don't need to chase anyone's talent.
You don't need to reject, hide, and doubt your gifts.
You don't need to look down on your body.

Let go of the imposed constructs and choose the life that creates happiness for you. You are the woman or man of your dreams. No one can take you away from you!

"Bag lady you gone hurt your back
Dragging all them bags like that
I guess nobody ever told you
All you must hold onto, is you, is you, is you..."
— Erykah Badu

Dragging around bags of unworthiness, judgement, shame, blame, and guilt will break your back. How do you let go of the baggage that stops you from seeing the beauty of you? How do you let go of pain, blame, guilt, shame? You have to be willing to look at everything you create and be present with it without running away.

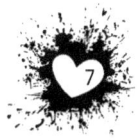

Running is always easy...

It's so easy to distract yourself with excess food, TV, exercise, sex, social media; to bypass the gifts you've created. This only further creates more blame, judgement, shame, and regret.

Being willing to look at everything destroys the control any situation has over you — being willing to look at what you create changes things.

What does it mean to look at things?

Be present with what is, without judgement. Being present provides the space for you to receive awareness of what it would take to change things. In some cases, you become aware that the stuff you've been holding onto isn't even yours, you just took it on because it seemed so real and true that you thought you owned it.

Awareness creates the space to ask questions...

If this is not mine, who does it belong to? This question, who does it belong to, doesn't require you to figure out who it belongs to. The question creates the space for a different possibility to emerge.

Notice how light you feel when you bring up all the garbage, blame, shame, guilt, judgement and ask who does this belong to? In the space of the question, lies freedom.

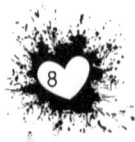

Blame and shame are designed to distract you from receiving the beauty and gift that is you. When you are blaming and guilting, you cannot perceive and receive you. When you are blaming and guilting, only more blame and guilt shows up.

There are many distractors designed to keep you from truly knowing how incredible and talented you are. Never be afraid of what you create — no matter how bad or ugly it may seem. You are greater than anything you create, and you have the power to change anything — this is one of your super powers.

You can change anything...

Once you realize that you are beautifully imperfect, nothing can take you away from you. All you must hold onto, is you, is you, is you.

> *"Gratitude for you changes everything."*
> — Gary Douglas

What would it be like to wake up each day in gratitude, aware of the precious gift that is before you — YOU?

We take ourselves for granted...

There are so many things we do and be for others: nurturer, creator of business and money, doctor, executive chef, lawyer, designer, negotiator, healer, lover, friend, miracle

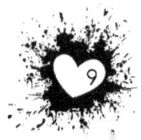

worker, consultant, accountant, editor, psychologist, advisor. All these are roles you may jump in and out of in a single 24 hours.

The amount of value you bring to the world cannot be measured. Your value is infinite!

Yet somehow we still seek validation and acknowledgement from others...

Seeking validation — waiting for someone to say...

Yes, you did a good job
Yes, you deserve a raise
Yes, you deserve me as your client
Yes, I will finally choose you
Yes, I will choose to marry you
Yes, I will choose to be in a relationship with you

... never knowing that you are the choosing one.

Being the choosing one is when you have no point of view of what a client thinks of you. It's when you choose to work with a client or not.

Being the choosing one doesn't require waiting to be chosen in a relationship. If you choose to be with me cool, and if you choose not to be, I wish you well.

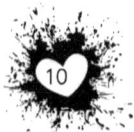

The choosing one doesn't wait for people to choose them...

If you're constantly waiting to be chosen, constantly seeking validation, you won't be able to see your own worth. Not seeing your own worth, you are constantly running, questioning, and wondering: "Am I good enough?" "Why don't they like me?" "Why won't he or she love me?" These are questions of doubt you wouldn't consider if you truly had gratitude for who you are; if you truly knew how valuable you are.

How do you cultivate gratitude for you?

Say to yourself 10 times in the morning and 10 times at night, "I am grateful for me, I am grateful for me, I am grateful for me, I am grateful for me, I am grateful for me, I am grateful for me, I am grateful for me, I am grateful for me, I am grateful for me, I am grateful for me."

Choose to be grateful for you every day until you are, until you feel gratitude for you in every molecule of your being. Stop waiting to be chosen. You are the choosing one.

Do not judge you; judgement and gratitude cannot exist at the same time. Instead, acknowledge you, acknowledge what you create, and acknowledge what you are creating.

What can you acknowledge about you every day?

I once read a powerful word on beauty, gratitude, and value; it goes like this:

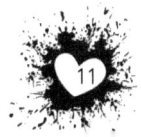

"I will tell you, my daughter
of your worth
not your beauty
every day. (your beauty is a given. every being is born
   beautiful).
knowing your worth
can save your life.
raising you on beauty alone
you will be starved.
you will be raw.
you will be weak.
an easy stomach.
always in need of someone telling you how beautiful
   you are."
— Nayyirah Waheed

What is one thing you can be grateful for, for you today?
Gratitude is potent — gratitude for you changes everything.

*"There was once a girl who doubted everything about her, when
she became a woman, a mother, a wife, in her 40th year of living,
she finally let go of all the BS. She let go of the lies that reigned in
her kingdom. She started adoring herself and living her life as a
celebration."* — Grace Engel

Creating your life and asking for what you truly desire is one
of the greatest gifts you can give yourself. I teach a course
called Creator of Magnitude, what do you desire to create?
Seeing participants take this class and 'get it,' is a precious
experience for me as a facilitator.

I've had a number of teens join this class and 'get it' in a
different way than adults. Teens are instant creators once
they're acknowledged for the magic they already are.

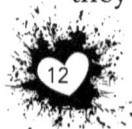

In your life — once you know that you can ask for what you truly desire, create it, and receive it — a whole new world is uncovered for you.

If there are areas in your life where you struggle, feel stuck, experience lack, self-doubt, pain, anger, rage, take a look at what it is that you've been unwilling to create. Your rage, pain, and anger may mask your unwillingness to honor you as a creator of magnitude.

> You must honor you as a creator.
> You must honor your creations and bring them out in the world.
> You must be willing to out-create yourself.

You will know your beauty once you acknowledge you as a creator. Your inner and outer beauty will radiate. Everything around you will contribute to you when you commit to creating your life.

Once the mountain of lies and BS that you have believed about what it takes to create your life, once these lies are exposed and rise to the surface - the lies will melt, the lies will dissolve, the lies will be destroyed.

You become a vibrational match to what you desire to create, and you will actualize your reality!

When she let go of the lies that reigned in her kingdom, she started adoring herself, living and creating the life she knew was possible.

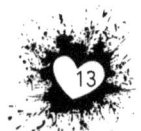

About the Author

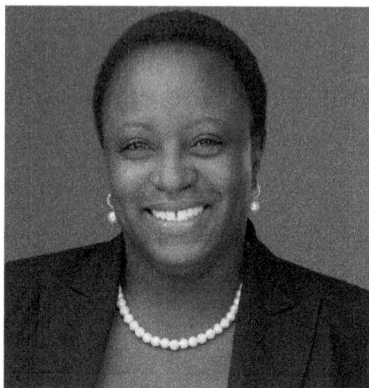

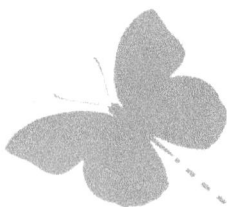

Grace Engel

Grace Engel is the creator and founder of Create with Ease. She works with clients facilitating them to walk in their power and create the life they know is possible. She is a facilitator of greater possibilities. She offers private coaching, local workshops, and online courses for those looking to create the life they have always known to be possible but haven't yet achieved. Grace works with teenagers assisting them to step into their potency and create beyond what they could only have imagined. Grace also offers Conscious Leadership workshops for corporations and organizations that inspires teams to create, and institute, in a different way that generates business growth and sustainability. She is also the host of The Create with Ease podcast.

You can find Grace here:
www.createwithease.com
www.facebook.com/BeBlissfulliving
@createwithease on Instagram
@creategreater on Twitter

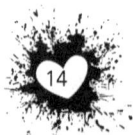

Chapter 2

The Day I Became Aware That "I Am Beauty"

Sarah Grandinetti & Cassy Summers

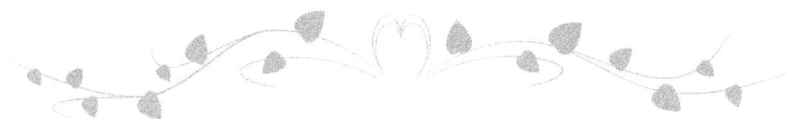

If you knew, without a doubt, the gift of the beauty of you, inside and out, would self-love be the side effect?

Self-Love

What does it even mean to love yourself? This is a question that seems to be elusive to most. Does it mean putting yourself before others? Does it mean judging yourself as perfect? Or does it mean loving yourself despite your imperfections?

What if it *could* mean something totally beyond all of that? What if loving yourself is a space of never making yourself wrong, never making yourself right and being in a continual forward motion of gratitude and acknowledgement for

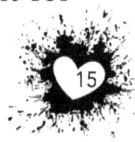

YOU? What would be different in your life if you knew without any doubt that you are one of the greatest gifts to this planet and you never had to prove it?

Self-love is not something outside of you. It's not something that comes after you are acknowledged, heard, or seen. It is a gift only you can give yourself.

The Ultimate Cake

You are an ingredient to a recipe you may not have yet acknowledged. You see, the moment you came into this world in the body that you occupy, you changed it. Yep, the whole world. Now, that may seem like an exaggeration, or an impossibility... but, does it actually create a lightness in your world?

SIDE NOTE & BEST KEPT SECRET OF THE UNIVERSE:

That which is true for you will always make you lighter that which is not true for you will make you heavier.

Ok, where were we? Right! The gift of YOU!

Have you ever made a cake from scratch? The first thing you need to do is get the ingredients together. You measure them out and add them to big bowl and start mixing. You eventually bake the yummy creation. The deliciousness starts to permeate the air around you and your mouth begins to water. The timer goes off and the excitement peaks! You

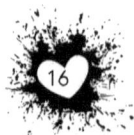

add the icing, fruit, or whatever mouthwatering topping you desire. Voila! You have a cake!

Now, what if you had forgotten the salt or baking powder? What if a key ingredient wasn't added to the cake? Would it still taste the same? Or even rise?

You are a key ingredient. Your presence on this planet changes the whole creation of it.

So, we are very glad you are here.

Our Self-Love Creation

Whether you were given this book as a gift or chose it from a search on the internet, you're more than likely reading it because you were aware of a possibility. That possibility may be to expand the self-love you already possess or to find it for the first time. Either way, we both know what it's like to follow the energy of a possibility, open to what it might create.

A few years ago, we had an awareness of a possibility. We had no idea where it would take us or what it would create for our business, but we knew we had to choose it. We were about to facilitate our first class together and in order to put ourselves out there and engage with people, we chose to create a 30-Day challenge on Facebook. We chose to do it around physical beauty and invite people to get out of the judgement that shows up when we choose to put any of our attention there. We were aware that somewhere it's

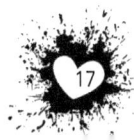

been accepted and deemed right and good if one works on their "inner self" but the minute someone wants to celebrate their beautiful body, it becomes a judgeable offense. So we created 30 challenges involving everything from "post a picture of your hands and share what you're grateful for with your hands' to "Write a letter to your teenage self and tell you what you wish you knew about your beauty". We called the challenge #IAmBeauty. It was the very first day of the challenge that we realized that we hadn't just created another 30-Day Challenge... we had created a Movement.

An Invitation to The Movement

What started out as a fun Facebook challenge, turned into a life changing movement that then asked to be classes held all around the world.

What we have seen show up in these challenges and classes are people of all shapes, colors, ages and sizes being courageous with their beauty, choosing communion and oneness while dynamically having each other's back.

IamBeauty is about celebrating beauty in all of its uniqueness. There are workshops all over the world that ask you to look at the "beauty within" and what we have noticed is that people have been seeing the celebration of their outer beauty as a wrongness and we are here to change that!

What if claiming your own physical beauty carried no separation but instead created a space to celebrate all beauty in its incomparable glory?

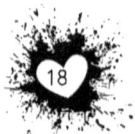

Our gift to you is a page from the manual that we affectionately call **The Starter Kit.** In this chapter, we would like to explore each step with you.

The
#IAmBeauty
Starter Kit

Step #1
Before your feet hit the floor every morning say 10×s
"All of Life Comes to me with Ease Joy and Glory"

Notice that this mantra doesn't say "some things in life" or "the good things in life", it says ALL of life, ladies and gentlemen. What does that mean? It means that you can choose to have Ease, Joy and Glory... even in the most difficult times of your life. The thing is, that's not what we're taught. We are taught that life is hard; something we have to deal with; something we just try not to screw up too bad. We are suggesting that there's something else possible by loving YOU enough to start each day with this mantra!

Step #2
Choose a question, any question, to play with that day.

The power of a question is like the magic wand you had all along and didn't even know it... like Dorothy and her ruby slippers in the movie, *Wizard of Oz*. If you are looking for ways to start on the Self-love Journey, you must start asking more questions. It's the conclusions about who you be, how you be, why you be, and where you be, that

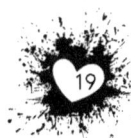

probably contributed to you ever falling out of love with you! Somewhere, at some point in time, a judgement that was cast at you stuck. It probably stuck, like it does for all of us, because we make the judgement real... more real than what we know to be true about us. This is where the all mighty question comes in and saves the day!! If you're drowning in the heaviness of judgement or conclusion, the question is your lifesaver! *"What else is possible here that I haven't considered?"*

"What's right about this (or me) that I'm not getting?"

"How does it get any better than this?"

These are all great questions to play with when you're in a funk.

Every morning start your day with the energy of a question. This puts you into the creation of your life right away. When you're creating your life, it's really hard to not possess self-love and gratitude for YOU, they seem to go hand in hand.

One of our favorite questions is:

"Universe, will you show me something beautiful about me today?"

Step #3

Move your body. Take a moment and breathe with it. Touch it kindly.

Invite gratitude for the Beauty of your body.

Being present with your body every morning can be the gift of awakening your senses and starting your day WITH your body in a truly dynamic way.

Here is an exercise you can do every morning:

As you begin to stir awake allow your attention to fall upon your entire body, from the top of your head down to your sweet toes. Feel the bed under you, feel your sheets, your clothes touching you.

Begin to stretch a little or a lot, bringing life to your muscles and warmth and fluid to your joints. Notice what is going on with your body now. If it could talk, what would your body say to you?

Now breathe. Become aware of your amazing lungs from the bottom all the way to the top. Without changing anything, notice the rhythm of the breath you already have. Does your breath sit high in your chest low towards your belly? Just notice. Now, with your attention present, take in a large slow breath, expanding your lungs as far as they would like to go. Breathe with your body now. In and out, in and out. Let your body set the pace. Do you notice the sense of peace available? Is your body grateful for these moments of attention?

Touch. If your body was the most precious and seductive thing you knew, how would you touch it? How would it like to be touched? Begin gently touching your skin. Where does your body desire to be touched? You may want to massage, or stroke, or have a feather touch. Explore this.

Would you be willing to touch even the places that you are in judgement of? If yes, then when you touch those places ask to increase the level of kindness in your touch. Perhaps

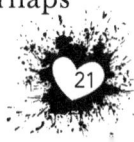

21

with more kindness then you've ever been touched with before.

Take another conscious breath as you move through this, touching, breathing and releasing judgment. Explore the possibilities of your body being a beautiful creation.

Say out loud "I Am Beauty."

Step #4

Each day, for a minimum of 1 minute, stand in front of a mirror and gaze into your own eyes.

Connect with you. What do you see behind those eyes? Would you be willing to allow your judgements of the person looking back at you to begin to wash away?

This little exercise is a doozy! You think it's nothing. You think, "I look at myself in the mirror every day!" Ya, well, you may be looking at the exterior and how your clothes look and if your hair is in place, but not many of us are looking into our own eyes. It can be very vulnerable if you'll allow for it. You will become aware of that person looking back at you that just desires to be loved and accepted... and that the person they want that from the most is you! You will see the kindness behind those eyes that has been desiring to come play even more. You might see the childlike wonder that you used to create your life with, gazing back at you. The pain that those beautiful eyes have shed tears over may rise up and expose itself. Whatever the experience you have from

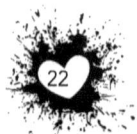

this exercise, the more you do it, the more you will find the adoration of YOU showing up! Intimacy with yourself is a big component to any love... and self-love is no different.

Step #5

Pick something about your body that you are in judgement of and for a minimum of 5 minutes a day pull up the energy of that judgment and repeat (out loud or in your head) "interesting point of view I have this point of view" over and over until you perceive a shift.

Repeat this process with a new body part as needed.

Now you may be wondering.... how is saying *"interesting point of view I have this point of view"* going to expand or create self-love? Well, let us tell you! Every single judgment you have about you and your body is just something you have decided to believe. Something you were told or shown, something you bought from your parents, or something this reality imposed on you. But what if you didn't have to believe any of it anymore?

What if you took this solid thing we call judgment (which is anything you make right or wrong) and you turned it into just an interesting point of view? Seems less intense than a judgment doesn't it? It's just an interesting point of view.

Each time you say it aloud you are turning the "real" solid judgments into something that is lighter and less significant. It's just... Interesting. and eventually your point of view about

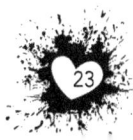

you may even become uninteresting. Don't take our word for it though, try it yourself!

Loving YOU enough

What if you loved yourself enough to do these exercises?

What does it take to fall in love with yourself?

Well, truly you are the only one that can answer that, but now you are equipped with some great tools to explore this possibility with.

If you can get to a place of knowing and acknowledging the contribution you truly are, then you will have you and if you have you, it's much easier to choose to love you!

You see, there is something that is so beautiful about YOU. Something no one else has.

You don't have to find it, define it, or prove it.

It's already there.... you just have to allow yourself to see it.

You are beauty.

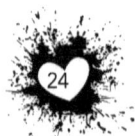

About the Authors

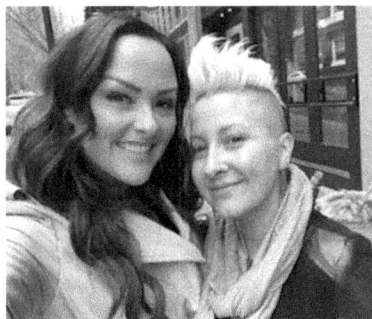

Sarah Grandinetti
Cassy Summers

Sarah Grandinetti and Cassy Summers, better known as "Sassy," are changing the way we see beauty. While sharing the energy of oneness as a possibility, they infuse their "THIS IS YOUR TRIBE" mantra in all of their creations. And that is what showed up in the #IamBeauty Movement a Tribe like no other. People go from feeling alone and disconnected to not only knowing that there are others out there that have their back but also that they desire to celebrate them. Sassy plays with this is in such a unique way in all of their classes, but the greatest way is the how they demonstrate it by having the back of each class participant supporting them to dive into their vulnerability and look at the places within themselves. With each their own unique gifts, together they are catalysts for change for whomever is in their wake.

Neither can be defined by their stats: both Access Conscious Certified Facilitators Sarah, salon owner, Marketing Wizard, mother of four, married for 15 years and Cassy, body worker,

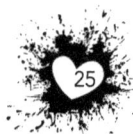

single mother of two and Creative Content Producer. Instead, these two women, upon meeting them, will be remembered by their out of the box facilitation to create MORE in everyone's lives they touch.

Sarah has a sterling knack for analogy; her storytelling pulls you in and you are held through all the turns until you arrive at the awareness at the mountain top of your own knowing.

Cassy is an exquisite mover of energy. Her perception is incomparable; the energy pulls she leads, if you are lucky enough to be present, leave you KNOWING you also can perceive and move energy.

So, put these two in the same room, and they are about to launch your life beyond your imagination.

www.iambeauty.space
https://www.sarahgrandinetti.com
www.curiousuniverse.ca

Facebook:
https://www.facebook.com/thejoyofsassy/
https://www.facebook.com/TheIAmBeautyMovement/?ref=br_rs
https://www.facebook.com/
TheIAmBeautyMovement/?ref=aymt_homepage_panel
https://www.facebook.com/AccessCassySummers/
https://www.facebook.com/sarahgrandinettiCF/

Instagram:
https://www.instagram.com/iambeauty_movement
https://www.instagram.com/asassyproduction
https://www.instagram.com/cassysummers

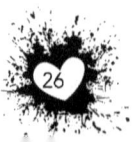

Chapter 3

My Journey of Self-Love, Trust and Healing

Tracey Chew

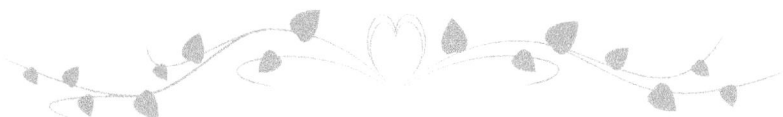

I am five years old sitting on a stool in my Nana's kitchen, listening to my mom argue with my dad on the phone. He left that day without saying good-bye. He disappeared and I did not see him again until 18 years later when I was 23 years old and graduating from college. I was shocked to find out he was alive; and devastated to learn that he had no remorse about abandoning us.

My self-love journey started with dramatic events at a young age, and it has had many ups and downs as I learned how to follow my heart while dealing with loss, broken trust and chronic illness. In response to challenges in my life, I did not trust others very easily. I became a keen observer of

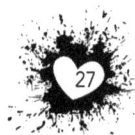

myself and others in order to ensure that I was safe. Broken trust became a core issue underlying many of my health and relationship challenges. I desperately sought health and happiness, but they were difficult to achieve. Like a dog chasing its tail, what I was seeking was within me, not outside of me. It took many years, but eventually I discovered the information I needed to heal my body, calm my mind, and love myself unconditionally.

Paying Attention

I was often sick and stressed as a child. As I grew up, I searched for health and happiness, and I began a long journey of self-discovery that had a surprise ending. In searching for the cause and cure for my symptoms, I discovered that I was both the cause and the cure. WHAT?! While trying to fix my broken body, I learned to calm my mind and stop doing the things that were stressing out my body. This allowed my body to heal more easily, and I have been living a much happier and healthier life ever since. I learned to pay attention to patterns and notice the core issue underlying my health and relationship challenges. My core issue was broken trust and it started when I was very young: first with my dad leaving, and then in a car accident that I will never forget.

I was six years old and my Mom and two younger brothers and I lived with another Mom and her three kids that were the same ages as us. The two girls and I would walk home from school every day. One day, they were both sent home early because they were sick. I only had to walk a few blocks

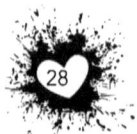

to reach my house and I was not afraid to do it by myself. I remember coming up to a stop sign and swinging around the pole. I saw a blue car approaching and I waited for the car to stop. The woman driver stopped, looked into her rear view mirror, and motioned for me to walk across the street. I stepped into the street and then stepped back onto the curb. I motioned for her to go first, and she impatiently waved her hands, motioning for me to cross first. I went, and then she drove over me. It was a hit and run. Miraculously, the car passed over me without the tires hitting my body. In a panic, I tried to get up while I was still underneath the car, and I gouged my head on something that cut into my scalp. I was able to get up by myself. By the time I got out of the street and fell to the curb, strangers were caring for me. When the ambulance driver came, I was not crying. I was spitting up blood and begging to go home.

Observing My Reactions

This event set the stage for me to develop very mixed feelings about people; and limited my ability to trust them. Although I grew up feeling that there are good people in the world who will help me, I also saw evidence that I cannot trust everyone to follow the rules, and that people might hurt me. As a defense, I became hyper vigilant and a keen observer of people. I falsely concluded that I needed to do more to earn people's trust, which would make me feel loved and safe. I became the family peace maker, good girl, and good student. I was everyone's little helper and I thrived on their approval. Receiving an A- grade was barely acceptable for me. I was trying to prove my worth, measure up, control

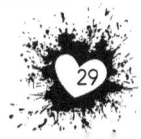

my behavior, and influence the reactions of others, so that people would like me and help me feel safe. I have lived my whole life with a very limiting belief that "I am not enough."

Soon after the car accident, I started to suffer chronic allergies and sinus infections. I was seven years old when the doctor put me on antibiotics for the first time. I developed a pattern of seasonal allergies that quickly progressed into sinus and bronchial infections. Every year, for decades, I consumed boxes of pills and cough medicine every few weeks, and antibiotics four times a year. I wanted good health at any cost, and I popped pills at the first sign of illness; but I abused Western medicine to the point where it lost effectiveness. For three decades, I was stuck in a cycle of feeling betrayed, discouraged, frustrated, scared and desperate because of my body's symptoms and their frequent occurrence.

As these efforts failed to help, I became curious and open to experimenting with all forms of eastern medicine, energy healing, and psychic clearing. I've had a wonderful adventure learning about the energy of our thoughts and emotions, and the ability of the mind to create or disrupt health in the body. Through this exploration, I learned that my negative feelings were adding stress to my hyper-sensitive immune system and compounding the problem. My life changed for the better once I learned to meditate.

Finding Peace

As soon as I heard my friend tell me about his experience at the Vipassana 10-day silent meditation retreat, I knew

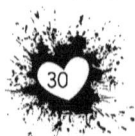

that I wanted to do it. The hairs stood up on my arms and I knew this was my body's signal to pay attention. I had never meditated before, and I wasn't sure I could sit still and be in silence all day, but I gave it my best shot. The first nine days were painful. I was uncomfortable sitting for so long, and my back felt like someone was dragging a knife down my spine. I got through it, and I was rewarded on the last day with an amazing experience. Very spontaneously, my brain was flooded with images of people dressed from all over the world, in vivid color as if they were right in front of me. I felt like I had tapped into some sort of cosmic National Geographic TV channel. It made such an impression, that I committed to doing Vipassana meditation two hours a day for the next year.

I was in my mid-30's and my commitment to meditate changed my life in a big way: I rearranged my schedule, reset my priorities, and I would slip into the back room at parties in order to meditate. The pay-off was that meditation helped me transform into a better person. I was aware of my thoughts, feelings and intuition. I was in tune with my body and I could manage my emotions. However, I was still suffering with chronic sinus infections and treating them with antibiotics. I was disciplined in doing everything I could to be healthy, but it was not working. Then a friend invited me to go camping with her and that trip led to a series of events that changed my health and my life forever.

Changing My Life

While I was practicing Vipassana, I shared an apartment in San Francisco with two friends and one of them liked to

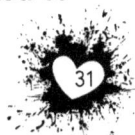

meditate. She invited me to go camping with her. While I was sitting on a rock in a shallow area of the river, I imagined playing there with my cousin's two boys who were seven and nine years old. I had not seen them in over a year, but I could imagine them playing in this river. The desire was so strong that I asked my cousin for permission to fly them up from San Diego to take them camping. I was single, with no experience taking care of children for a week on my own, but graciously, my cousin let me do it. Within the first 24 hours of camping, I met the man that I would marry and his two children. His son was the age of my two young cousins. I would not have talked to them, if not for my cousins who wanted to play with this man's son.

Meditation increased my ability to listen to my body and follow my heart. When I did that, everything changed quickly. Within a year, I changed jobs, moved to a new city, got married, became a step-mom, and stopped the cycle of chronic illness.

Healing with Awareness

After the first year of being married, I experienced more health and less sickness. I only needed antibiotics once a year instead of four times a year. At first, I attributed my improved health to the healing power of love and being happy. However, my marriage ended after 11 years, and I did not revert back to having chronic illness. My body had changed over the course of my marriage. I trusted my husband completely and this was a surprise catalyst for healing my body. With my ability to trust and feel loved,

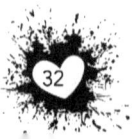

my body was able relax, become more resilient to stress and more capable of staying healthy. The radical change in my body opened my eyes to the power of my mind to affect my health; and showed me how important it is to heal my core issue of broken trust.

After my divorce, I made a conscious effort to pay attention to my mental health, and change negative habits impacting my body. I voraciously studied everything I could find pertaining to how the mind affects the body, and vice versa. I became skilled at using the tools and eventually, I became a professional life coach and taught others to use them as well. After attending dozens of workshops, I gained the most insight and inspiration from these leaders: Louise Hay, Bruce Lipton, The HeartMath Institute, and Marissa Peer. I am especially grateful to John Assaraf for compiling knowledge from the best brain scientists to help people change their habits and improve their outcomes. As a direct result of all that I have learned and experienced, I have developed a strong belief that I can rebuild my body and rewire my brain to be positive and happier; and every day, I am living in that truth.

My health depends on supporting my immune system and managing thoughts that create anxiety and stress. My intuition told me that I had to stop pushing myself past my physical limits. I had to learn to say no and risk disappointing others. I had to manage the anxiety about not being good enough and not being able to trust others. I had to stop over-thinking, over-doing, and staying up too late working because the chronic stress and nervousness made my immune system over reactive.

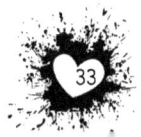

Mindfulness tools have helped calm my mind, ease my anxiety, and reduce my symptoms. However, a lot of damage was done over the years, and now I am living with an autoimmune disorder called Hashimotos. I am better equipped to handle this challenge today than I would have been 15 years ago. I accept the condition as a part of my life. I do very simple practices based in loving kindness that help relieve symptoms and allow me to live in peace with the disorder. Mindfulness and meditation continue to be my best defenses against any challenge in my life.

Rewiring My Brain

One of the many gifts of my self-love and healing journey, is the discovery of science-based techniques that can change my brain if I practice them consistently. I learned one from training with Marissa Peer that worked really well for me and my clients. It involves repeating the phrase "I AM ENOUGH" while looking into your eyes, in the mirror. At first, it brought tears to my eyes, and I could feel the power of this phrase. I invited my clients to join me to do an "I AM ENOUGH" challenge for 40 days saying this phrase for 40 times a day. Everyone felt better at the end of the challenge. I still smile when I think of one woman who did it for 3 months. At first, she couldn't say the words without crying. It took her 30 minutes a day to get through the 40 repetitions. She could barely look in the mirror much less say the words because she was deeply connected to the pain and shame from her marriage ending against her will. Her emotions were disrupting her work and she was willing to try this technique to feel better. She was consistent with

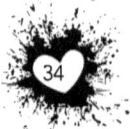

saying the phrase, and it got easier with time. By the end of the first month, she was stronger. By the end of the third month, the thought of her ex-husband no longer hurt her, and she started living a happier life.

I believe it is true that no one can love you better than yourself. My client's husband could never give her what she gave to herself by looking into her own eyes, repeating I AM ENOUGH, and believing it. Like my client, I have started healing my psychic and emotional wounds by looking into the mirror and affirming myself. Self-love is a journey that takes time, but I have deliberately enhanced it by practicing certain techniques.

Practicing Daily

Life is a series of choices, and my life gets better when I choose to focus on being loving to myself and taking care of my body. I use simple tools to create more peace and recover quickly when I am upset. If I am having any negative reactions in my relationships, then I look to see if my core issue about trust is influencing my perceptions in a negative way. I am not perfect. I make regrettable choices and I get upset. The difference now, is that they happen with less frequency and impact, and I handle them with greater compassion and understanding.

These are the four tools that I use every day:

1. MAKE A CHOICE of how I want to be. I choose to be loving and kind. This mindset guides my actions throughout the day.

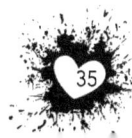

2. MINDFULNESS allows me to pause, check in, and notice what I feel, and what I need to be healthy and happy. Mindfulness helps me pay attention and gives me an opportunity to choose wisely. Otherwise, I slip back into old habits.

3. MEDITATION is healing. It helps me listen to my intuition and pay attention to the sensations in my body that is always communicating with me for my own good. Meditation helps me have more self-awareness and peace.

4. MANTRAS like "I AM ENOUGH" can be programmed into my brain with consistent daily repetition. For example, after eight years of programing "Tracey I Love You" into my brain, it is now the first thing I hear in the morning when I wake up. It's a beautiful and affirming way to start the day.

Believing I Am Loveable

"You can't love another until you learn to love yourself," I heard this phrase growing up, and I believe it is true. My self-love journey led me to realize that I am the one who can love myself best; and my mind affects my experience of health and happiness. Loving myself is a daily choice followed by a commitment to take actions that make me feel that way. Every day I pause to check-in and notice how I am feeling, so that I can change my perspective in order to feel better. I am intentionally kind, compassionate and loving with myself, and I let go of judgement and self-criticism as much as possible. The more compassionate I can be, the more tolerant I become of my imperfections and mistakes. The more I like myself, the more I love myself. The more

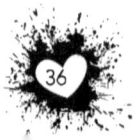

I do this, the easier it is for me to trust and love others unconditionally, because I don't need or expect anything in return. I fulfill my own needs for feeling safe and loved.

Living in Love

We all know that life is hard and full of challenges, frustrations, disappointments and tragedies. There are many things that I cannot control, even within my own body, and my best defense has been to accept what is happening in the moment with compassion. Each relationship and event in my journey, helps me learn about myself so I can make better choices to be healthy and happy. In hindsight, I can identify bad choices that I have made, but I don't regret them. These experiences remind me that I am resilient and capable of changing for the better. I know that I can overcome anything with grace and good humor. I live and learn from my mistakes. The more I pay attention to my thoughts and feelings, the more opportunities I have to make good choices. Can you imagine what our world would be like if we all did this?

Today I live with the mindset and energy of love. If you look at my life now, compared to where I started my journey, I am living a Cinderella story. Everything has changed for the better because I choose to pay attention, be mindful, be loving and kind in my thoughts and actions, and follow my heart. I wake up hearing the worlds "I love you, Tracey" in my own voice. I don't beat myself up when I make mistakes. I handle things that make me stressed with a lot more ease. I relate to my body as a friend and I don't push past my physical limits. I give my body what it needs to be healthy and energetic. I am grateful to live with the "Love of my Life" and we intentionally cultivate a loving relationship based in truth, trust, kindness and respect. We have created a beautiful home and meaningful relationships with kind neighbors, friends and family. I have a clear vision of what I want to be in my golden years, and I have a strategy and a plan to keep me on track to get there. It involves living one day at a time, one breath at a time, and with great self-awareness and compassion.

I wish you great success in your journey of self-awareness and self-love. I believe that I am loveable, and I am enough; and I wish for you to believe the same about yourself.

My last offering to you is a quote from Charlie Chaplin's Love Yourself Manifesto.

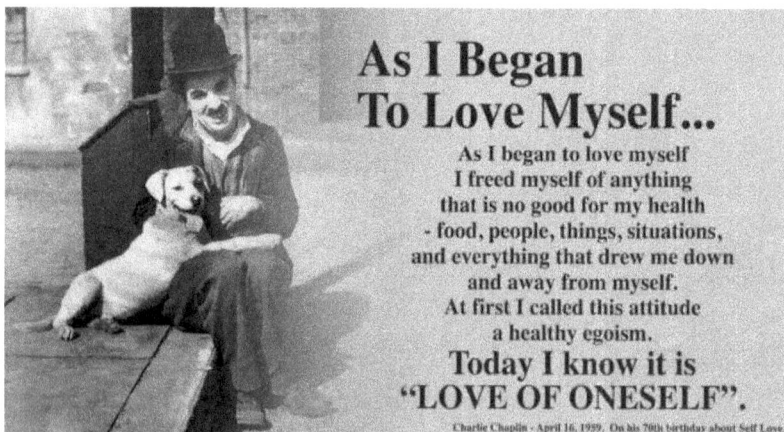

As I Began
To Love Myself...
As I began to love myself
I freed myself of anything
that is no good for my health
- food, people, things, situations,
and everything that drew me down
and away from myself.
At first I called this attitude
a healthy egoism.
Today I know it is
"LOVE OF ONESELF".
Charlie Chaplin - April 16, 1959. On his 70th birthday about Self Love.

https://understandingcompassion.com/articles/began-love-charlie-chaplin-beautiful-poem-self-love/

About the Author

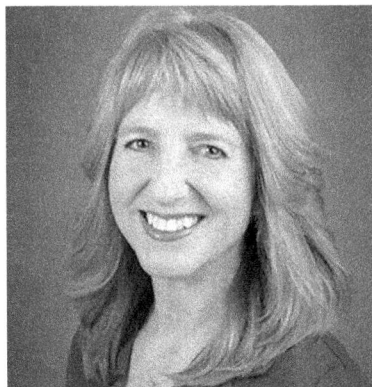

Tracey Chew

I am happily growing my own business, after retiring from 20 years of leadership in nonprofit housing services in the Bay Area of California. Since 2009, I have enjoyed providing leadership and mindfulness coaching to executives, influencing and enhancing their ability to become self-aware and mindful of their thoughts, emotions, and reactions to manage stress, and enhance productivity. I practice what I teach; and every day, I meditate; set an intention for loving kindness to govern all of my actions; pause throughout the day to assess how I am feeling and be proactive to keep feeling my best.

I am a Heart Ambassador and my future goals are to train United Nations representatives and high-level government leaders to use technologies developed by the Heart Math Institute to enhance self-awareness, mindfulness, and heart-based decision making. I am interested in teaching heart-based living to youth to influence the future leaders of our country to have disciplined

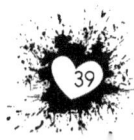

minds that are self-aware, self-regulating and responding to life's challenges with kindness and compassion.

In my personal time I enjoy meditating, hiking, gardening, dancing, road trips, wine tasting, camping, yoga, and learning everything I can about the influence of the mind and the heart in healing the body. I am a native of California and I currently live with the "Love of my Life" in San Jose.

I have a master's degree in Urban and Regional Planning from Virginia Tech; a BA. in Sociology from UCLA; and I am a certified Professional Life Coach, Neuro-Linguistic Practitioner, Self-Esteem Coach, and Trainer of the Ritberger Personality Method. I served four and a half years in the Peace Corps and I speak conversational Spanish.

Contact me at: tlc@traceychew.com
TLC Mindfulness Mentor Website: www.traceychew.com
https://www.facebook.com/tlcmindfulnessmentor/

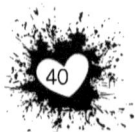

Chapter 4

Self-Love is Not Self-Sacrifice

DeAnna Lee (and guides)

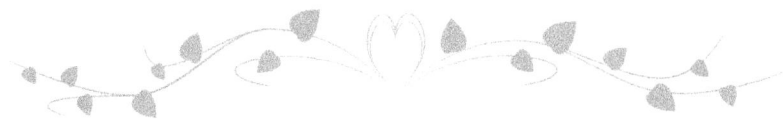

This is a transcript from a channeled session. DeAnna Lee, physical medium, channels wisdom from her guides. The messages are from spirit including those from Thomas Jefferson and others.

Thomas & Guides: You may call me Thomas. There will be more than one speaking with thee today.

Interviewer: Thank you Thomas.

Thomas & Guides: We understand that we are speaking about love and self-love. The first thing that many think of when thinking of self-love is sacrifice.

When they are thinking not of self-love, but of loving, they think of sacrifice. We would like to make a very pointed significant difference between sacrifice and love. Love never requires sacrifice. Self-love *is* loving others.

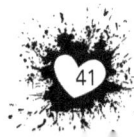

How could that be? Some will say how can that be? If I love myself, how can that be truly loving another? And we would want you to know that when you're honoring yourself, you're honoring source within you, your own being, and your own soul. That is an expression of source. That source and self are connected, inseparable. When one is honoring self and loving self, true self. Not Ego self, but what is in the heart, what is in the deepest part of the desiring. And in the heart that is where source speaks to thee. When thee love self from that place that is for the benefit of all. And it allows and frees others to go on their true paths as well. And in that process, there is no sacrifice involved. We assure thee that source does not know of sacrifice.

Source loves each one unconditionally, infinitely, and at all times. And that is not through sacrificing. That is through being source's self, source's expression of source's own being. And each person being of source in their true being. It is the same. It is like a universal law of source. It is a universal law of life that when one is acting from a place that is the creator of all of life.

That frees life to flow and each one to go on their own path and journey as they should. If a person is in the mindset that I must sacrifice to be loving, that is more a self-imposed idea. Do you understand?

Interviewer: Yeah, that really hits close to home yesterday. I got present to how it's hard sometimes to feed the kids. I feed them and then not me.

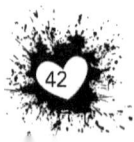

Thomas & Guides: Indeed. And it is not honoring them in the way that you would truly honor them as well. You are teaching at that moment that one of your family, namely you, are not as important as the rest of the family. That each is not equal. And in truth, each one in the family is as worthy of love as another. And that is what you would want to teach them as being loving to them. If the portions must be smaller, then so be it. No one will starve. There will be enough. Or perhaps it is that you are too busy and do not care for yourself.

Whatsoever the reason is, it's not good enough reason to not love yourself. And it's also not truly loving them. Do you understand why? Everyone here is here to teach each other. And each one comes truly from a high place of love for each other. It is that each one loves everyone here more than they are aware of. The whole purpose of coming is to join and love and teach one another.

They have come to teach you as well as you have come to teach them. Not just as a parent but in soul of the value and honor of each life. And the greatest gift you could give any other human being is to teach them the significance of loving themselves. That often also requires that one be courageous and brave as it is not an easy practice.

The courage to love yourself once again goes back to getting centered within self, asking self what self needs. And then having the courage to stand in that. With the intention and desire to be loving as well.

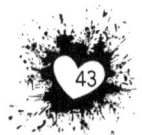

It is not I love myself more than I love another. It is that I love myself and all others as well.

I hold a balance in my heart for myself and everyone else that I love.

This seems to be the greatest difficulty for others to overcome. For individuals to overcome is this idea of sacrifice as become a part of loving. And it is just the opposite. Love never requires sacrifice. The only thing that is given up is those things that are not true. Everything that is not love may fall away. And only love stands supreme. It would be helpful to distinguish what's of source light and love and also comes from within your own being. And what is a false idea of love.

This is a practice and a process.

Thomas & Guides: I am so loving when we speak of loving. This is something that is not generated by the mind, it is of the heart. It is from the inner self. It is not a thought projection.

Love is a natural flow from your connection with source. Whether you are aware of it or not, does not matter. It is connected to source and allowing that to freely flow from self to others. One may choose to stand in that flow or to step out of it each day, and in moments when one is trying to decide what is loving and what isn't. And what would be the most loving thing to do.

One can have a check-off list of sorts to begin. And that is, am I making a sacrifice? If the answer is yes, then the

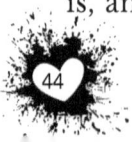

thought is a check that it is not love. Am I projecting from my mind what I think love is? One check that it is not love.

Am I standing within myself in my feelings? And my most inner self and wanting to express from that place wanting to allow love to flow through me to the situation or this being, this person. Then that is a check in, it is love and this I am wanting to and desiring to express. This check-list, if one goes through, they will be able to quickly come to what is and what isn't love. Then from that place of I have made my checklist, then we can see where you stand at that moment. If you stand truly in the intention and desire to love. Or if you're standing in the intention and desire to impose your own thought process of what love is onto the situation or to the person. And that would never be helpful to them, nor to you.

Go to that for a moment and think of it. And from that we could say I am one in the plus and two in the minus, and so I have a bit of work to do. What is the work I need to do to get to all positive and not any in the negative column to the best of my ability at this moment? And from that place then ask self again, what would be the most loving thing. And ask source what would be the most loving thing and allow that to flow through you. To the person or situation. And this may require something that you do not in your mind agree with or think is necessarily the right course of action. Then we have the courage to do it and then we have the trust that you are standing in your own truth and self-trusting yourself and trusting source.

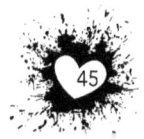

No Separation Between Self and Source

And we can even say at this moment that there is never a separation between the true self and source. But you do not need to think what would God do? That again, brings in the thought of what you think God would do? What your ideas of what God may be? And do rather than what God is and that again is in the negative column and does not added column for expressing the truth of love. It is the truth of love that we would have people begins to understand and live from. The idea of love is as there are many ideas here of what love is. There is the maternal love, paternal love, romantic love, friendship, and love, this distinguishing about love. And in truth it's all simply love. It is not all of these different names that are put on it. When you go to your own truth about how may I have the intention and desire to be the most loving being for myself. And each one that I can. And right away whatever comes, having the courage and trust to do that. Knowing in yourself that you are not separate from source. Once you do will be what are necessary for your growth and your path and that of the others as well. That is the trust

There are many steps in this process as one goes through it. It is not an easy practice to begin with. Some are further along in this practicing. We can move to that space of knowing within self-more quickly than others. That is a mount that also involves knowing oneself well enough to know the truth. One's true feelings, one's true own heart and being versus ones thought process. And whether one is clear with themselves or not. And everyone knows this

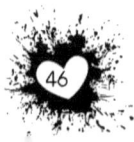

right away. This is an easy question for most people. If they will ask themselves, am I clear with myself, with my feelings and thoughts. Right away the answer will come, yes I am, or no, I'm not.

Thomas & Guides: Self-love, who is the self that I love. And many do not know. Many do not know who the self is. I would say that it is important that each one begin to have the journey of self-knowledge. And as each one does this, what they love will naturally come. Will quite just naturally come to them. What is love for them? Each one expresses this differently. As you are all unique in yourselves. Unique creations of source. What is love in your soul? And being. Take a difference direction or focus on another person. This is not a generalized, we all love in this certain way or not. It is getting to know self as well.

Thomas & Guides: So the journey of self-discovery and self-love is the greatest thing you can do in a lifetime. If you were to spend an entire lifetime learning this, it would be the greatest lifetime that you have ever had. As far as your own growth and development and also in being of service to others.

Interviewer: So I think I might be asking this for many, whose parents maybe said, you're good when you do good in school. Or you're good when you get a job or you're good when you have a thin body. Or you're good when you're this or that. That got very confusing because then it seemed like love was only when you were passing the test of some kind.

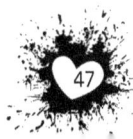

Can you speak to kind of raising consciousness beyond that? Or starting to love yourself even if you're not those things.

Thomas & Guides: Within this true self that is what we are speaking of self-discovery. What has caused me to feel unlovable? What has caused me to feel that I am worthy of love. Even that I am not worthy of love from others, but that I also am not worthy to love myself. This is the journey of self-discovery. And healing those aspects of self that I've felt unloved. And we would say that as there are many separations, as each separates loved into categories, here on the earth, as you were saying. Each one also separates parts of themselves within their own beings. I am not lovable because I am overweight. I am not lovable because I'm not smart enough. I'm not lovable because Mrs. Cook told me in my younger years that I couldn't read, write, speak correctly, or did not have proper writing skills. And on and on it goes that many have put these thoughts into each, every human being here has that thought. The journey of self-discovery is finding those places within self that do not feel lovable with courage and humbleness.

Strength standing with an open heart, embracing those things within self that they do not perceive as being lovable. As you yourself embrace those separated areas within self, they become whole.

Thomas & Guides: Have you heard the term compartmentalization?

Interviewer: Yes.

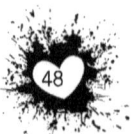

Thomas & Guides: In the mind, many have walls around. This is my work persona, this is my parenting persona. This is my place where I lock away thoughts that hurt me and caused me emotional pain. And there are many who have so many of these compartments within their own minds.

When one is separated within self, such a high degree has the individual locking their minds, putting away memories that are painful. Or the mind itself does not visit even is not whole as there are these separations within it. Really the idea of compartments is a good analogy to heal those separated parts of self. To begin this self-love journey as we were speaking of, how I can love myself if one does not know the self they love? Then love cannot flow to them. It becomes a chaotic energy or an energy that is not directed in a loving way. It adds to the difficulty rather than it is assisting. The first process can be an ongoing and sometimes life time process for some. To embrace those parts of self that are separated within their own beings. And how does one do this? The only a way to we to do this is to walk through it, to stand in the pain and allow it to stand in it, to allow the feelings of it. To get to the bottom of why a certain thought caused a certain feeling. And whether this is still fits or not.

And if it still feels like it fits, that means it is simply an unhealed part of self. It is part of self that needs your love that you have not loved this part of self.

Recognize those areas within self are areas that are in need of self-love. Those are areas that the individual themselves has pushed away within themselves. And these areas are in

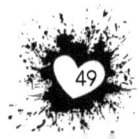

need of embracing, experiencing, and releasing. This is a bit of work. Is it not a surprise that you could take some a whole lifetime through this process? More a separation within themselves than others. Yet it applies to the most separated and the least. As each one has a degree of this or they would not be on the planet.

Interviewer: For some reason I'm being shown to ask about. I don't know why I am being asked this. So I'm just going to ask the question and then just do what you like. But if we feel moved to help like severely impoverished communities. Or we want to help those much less well off than ourselves. Or like I've always been driven to help like the very, the people who can't read. Or you know what I mean, like the very impoverished. Maybe talk a little bit about like where love comes in when we see people going through so much. Does that make sense?

Thomas & Guides: It is again a process. It is the understanding. If this comes from the heart, the true self, that I have this passion. You said passion. I have a passion to do this. That is love, passion is love. For you that would be self-love as well. If I see a brother on the streets who is in need, I have no passion for this and truly no desire, and then it is not self-love and demeans the other as well. Throwing a dollar in a bucket when I am not doing this because I have a love for this brother. But out of a sense of obligation would create an energy flow of anger. With a dollar that they are throwing in the bucket. They are throwing also a bucket full of anger at them as well. That could not be in spirit ever viewed as love. We are not suggesting that you do not help

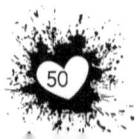

those that you see in need. We are distinguishing between what we are truly giving. Are they giving from love? If they are that is what the brother will receive. If you are giving out of obligation, then the brother will receive a very different energy that would not be love. Then so you are adding to their difficulty rather than lessening it.

That is why it's is so crucial for one who desires this path and not all do desire this path. And that is all right as well. But for those who do desire this path of self-love extend that to all in their lives. And this would it be something they would; each one must consider and think of as they go through their day. And with practice it becomes an instant knowing the thoughts may go through my mind. I would like to give that brother the dollar, yet my heart immediately feels that no, I do not really want to do it. But it is the socially right thing to do. And I will know instantly that what I am giving is not love. What I am giving is I am sharing a social obligation that I have no feeling about. Or feel angry about or feel like I do not care about. And that brother receives that information. It's not totally what you do share, it is what you choose not to share as well. We would also go back to really understanding this self-love from a perspective of self-healing. Of embracing self in every area that has separated itself. Have separated from within the own being.

As thee cannot be a whole expression of love if you have all of these places that one is stuck in separation. Separation and love do not go together. In any way and any form at any time. Separation is always separation and love is always inclusive. It is always whole. We would just want to be clear

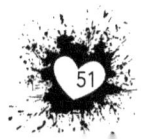

to everyone that desires this path that the first idea in self-love is to become non-separated within self. And as that occurs and less and less separation is walking about with your face on it, then you become more in line with universal laws. And Universal Energy and begin to be that flow of love. Your very presence begins to emanate that love. Then there is no thing that you must do except to show up. As it's becomes such a radiating energy that all of those around thee feel loved by your very presence.

When one is whole and stands holy in truth rather than the untruth of love. Then each one around them feels that. Everyone knows where thee stands at all times. Other brothers always feel whether you bring love or not or if you bring a mixture of love and self. Self-meaning separation, separate itself. Do thee understand?

Interviewer: These are things I know because we're also connected telepathically. So I am always able to perceive other people. Like I can see their bodies, I know where they're hurting. Like it's my body is shown what other beings are experiencing.

Thomas & Guides: Every brother here is as each one is from source. Everyone has the perception of the energy of another. We often tell each one that there is no hiding. And everyone thinks because I am in a separate body with a separate brain, I may somehow hide what my thoughts are. Are my intentions are or my desires or rather I am a clear channel of love or not. And thee may not hide this. Something that is either present or not. And everyone

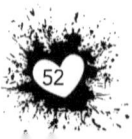

feels this to a certain degree from another person's energy. Whether it is through thoughts or just experiencing the way that they feel when they're around them. There are many forms of communication. In spirits, one learns as soon as they get to this side that they are an open book. And have always been an open book. Yet we're under the misguided impression that they were hidden somehow. Because they had a separate body or mind. And yet spirit always sees through that. And each one being spirits here sees through it as well. Of course it does vary in degrees.

We would say that love is always allowing. If one were to use Joshua or Jesus as it's known in his life, be allowed all others to be just as they were. He focused on his own being, his own connection with source. He did not focus on what others were doing. He focused on what he was doing. And when people are thinking, why does God allow this? Why does God allow that? If God loves me, why is this occurring? How could this occur if God loves me? And we would have each one understand that it is a misunderstanding of love. Love is holy allowing. As we go back to what we were saying earlier, love is also holy. Allowing oneself to allow oneself to be holy, who they are in truth. And going through and taking the fine tooth comb through the sections and parts of self that has kept aside the reason that that is so healing is because it is based on false ideas and thoughts of who you are. We would always want each one to only allow themselves to be just as they are. And to release those ideas and thoughts that are not of self. You do not come from self.

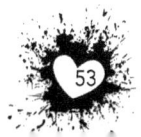

It's allowing only allowing for self and others and that this does not require sacrifice. Alright.

Thomas & Guides: Indeed. As this is a lifetime practice for the book, we would suggest that each one remember to stop and ask themselves. Am I acting on love through my true passion and desire? Or am I acting on sacrifice?

Interviewer: Perfect.

Thomas & Guides: Indeed.

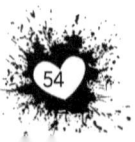

About the Author

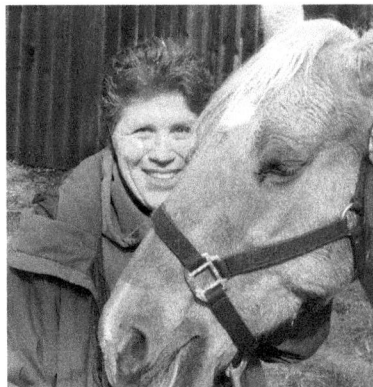

DeAnna Lee

DeAnna Lee lives in Colfax, California with three horses, dogs, a few goats, 15 love birds, her indoor piggy Pearl, and cats too. She has received messages from "her council" on the other side for more than 30 years, and channels these messages when asked.

DeAnna's first #1 bestselling book "I Have a New Dream" co-created with Erica Glessing included messages from the spirit of the late Dr. Martin Luther King, Jr. released on Martin Luther King Day 2019.

Find out more or sign up for a channeling session: FreetoAwaken.com.

Chapter 5

Self-Love

Dr. Kathleen McNulty

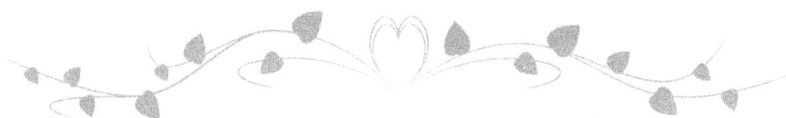

H ow is it that we love ourselves less than or very little? How is it that we don't take very good care of ourselves yet put others on pedestals?

What is Self-Love? Is Self-Love innate or something we learn or both. Can our ability to Self-Love be damaged? Our God self, the spark of the divinity within us is perfect and is Love. It is our human self that can become damaged and disfigured. Stand in front of a mirror and say:" I love myself".

Love is our innate state of being. Our divine nature is LOVE. It is our humanness and our human experiences here on earth that create separation. Love becomes dim and self-hatred and hatred of others develops. We feel we were "wronged". Our parents with their human limitations

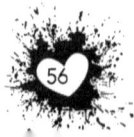

hurt our emotional bodies and self-hatred and/or loathing develops. "Others" harm us, threaten us, place fear in our hearts. These are all human created, human made. Divine LOVE can never be destroyed. Love is always within us.

Our human experiences here on earth challenge our spiritual growth. We can choose love or fear. Fear develops as others maim our physical bodies and our psyche. When we think of spiritual leaders such as Christ, Buddha, Mahammad and others; we learn that they separated the earthly experiences from themselves. They remained with the divine within them.

Loving ourselves is a spiritual challenge as we move forward to recognize the truth of our existence. There are many better (good) human beings on this earth than not. We need the love of others, good loving beings to assist in the healing of our damaged humanness. As this occurs, we can begin to love ourselves again and connect with the divine love within us. The passage to loving ourselves is a community process. A community can be two people or more. The extension of genuine love and care for the soul of another with understanding of the damage done to their human body, mind and emotion allows the healing process to begin. This opens our system to receiving new perceptions of the world (earth). As the mind considers these new perceptions, the human brain can create new neuronal pathways that adjust and realign our bodies to health and balance. We are readjusting to our natural state of self-love. Initially this may feel strange as in meeting yourself for the first time. Different behaviors will emerge such as not

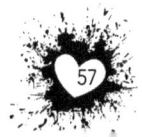

tolerating someone else's mistreatment of you whether that is with words or physical harm. You will elevate yourself in understanding that you are a child of the universe. You are deserving of all that is. You now accept compliments and graciously respect yourself as you offer respect to others. There are many pathways to self-love. The extension of love to others (those deserving of your love) lifts you even higher as you recognize each other's soul.

Self-love defines your internal world as a place of honor, a holy place. This internal view connects with the divine. Our bodies are temples for our spirit. Our spirit is one with the divine. As we heal our humanness, we recognize our holiness. It is also true that that which we have suffered as humans and healed are the avenues we've chosen for our soul's growth. This process assists in the development of empathy, a magnitude of understanding for the human condition and a doorway to heaven. Heaven is always there. It is our mortal existence here that clouds our vision and knowledge of our true origins.

Another path to self-love is through the connection with spirit and our loved ones who have passed over. Connecting with the sacred and asking for intervention for healing opens a portal for heaven to intervene and assist in healing our human ailments. The universe is omnipresent and ready to shower us with all that is needed. They can only intervene at our heartfelt genuine request. Expressing gratitude for all blessings we receive and for all that is and accepting responsibility for our part in the negative conditions on earth provides access to the abundance of healing that

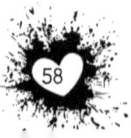

our minds and bodies require. Meditation and prayer are physical, mental states that transport our spirit to commune with God, the divine. As we engage in a regular practice of meditation and prayer, the very chemicals in our bodies and brains have the opportunity to change and produce healing chemicals which place us in a deep state of relaxation. This deep state of relaxation was always available to us. Somehow the damage we've suffered as humans initially create a resistance to this practice. Persistence is the best avenue to overcome this resistance.

Quiet your mind and sit in the stillness. As negative thoughts and or emotions arise, notice them and let them pass through your mind and exit. These are not the truth of you. Most likely negative thoughts and emotions are the product of others depositing their negativity into your vessel. You need not accept this as it doesn't belong to you. If right now you lack self-love, it is easier for others to "dump" their trash into your receptacle. Close the lid to your receptacle. Protect your mind body and energy field from others lower level health and lower level energy. They will seek to expunge their "garbage" to an open receptacle that seems willing to accept garbage. You are not a garbage container. Eliminate these dark low-level energies that only seek to bolster their egos as they are damaged and not seeking to heal. You can bless them and send them love and light for their own healing but DO NOT BECOME A RECEPTACLE for them.

Humans are at all different levels. Those of us who have awakened and seek to understand that we are spiritual

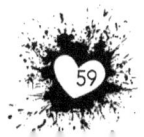

beings having a human experience, place themselves on a journey of self-love and understanding.

Practice seeing the light in others. Practice connecting soul to soul. However, be aware to practice with others who genuinely seek the divine as you do.

The journey to self-love is an honorable road, a spiritual road if you will. There are many holy people who care for the soul of others and extend a genuine healing path to self-love, self-care and spiritual growth.

Always remember who you are, you are a child of God no less than the sun and moon. You have a right to be here and deserve the power and love of God's healing grace. Allow the energy of love that is all around you to envelope you as you mediate and pray. This energy which all of earth is made of is God Source and available to us all. As you create a practice of stillness and connecting with the divine, remember to listen to your soul's whispering. These whisperings direct you toward your healing that needs to occur for your human healing. This human healing combined with spiritual understanding and knowledge creates a healthy internal atmosphere for your mind, body and soul. Self-love is the outcome.

May God surround you with peace. May you follow your soul's yearning. May you accept the abundance divine provides for you. May you eternally know we are all connected. Therefore, we create an energy of love that cannot be broken. Lean on your brother/sister to remember

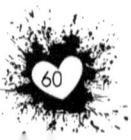

who you are. You are love, eternal love and heaven is closer than you think. Heaven is our breath and closer than our hearts.

Love yourself as God loves you.

Some journeys of healing that we came here to do are so vast and many. They are multilayered and create something like a mosaic. We are born to parents and families that we choose for our soul's growth. Often the parents and families we choose to be born into are psychologically damaged and place our human selves in an early life that sets us up for human emotional challenges. For example, one such healing story is of a middle-aged man who was born to a mother who "wanted a girl". She consistently told him this from a young age and told all her friends and relatives. His emotional body developed to believe he was an unworthy human being, low self-esteem and that he couldn't say no to authority figures as his mother was also emotionally absent and distant from him. He was horribly abused physically, sexually and emotionally by middle school coaches. These men brought their male friends and a few other young boys and abused them for years. By the time I sat with now middle-aged man, he was broken. A turning point in our weekly meetings together was when I kept repeating to him: "This wasn't your fault". He responded each time: "Yes, it was my fault. I'm defected. I could've said no." He had shared with me multiple times how his mother never allowed him to say "no" ever. I reminded him of this and attempted to remove this from his psyche as I offered my ego strength for him to lean on. He felt my compassion and directed healing

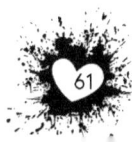

words in community. This same evening, I sat across from him and screamed at God in my head. I was screaming so loud in my head that I thought he would see my tears for his suffering. "God, I wasn't there when these terrible things were done to this man, your child!!!! YOU WERE!!!! Please heal him NOW!!!"

The next day I received a phone call from this middle-aged man whom I met with weekly for months. He stated ion the phone to me: "It wasn't my fault! It wasn't my fault! It wasn't my fault!" He was relieved, grateful and crying. He shared with me that the next morning when he picked up the newspaper, the front page had a picture of four men being arrested and handcuffed by the police and placed in police cars as they were caught abusing young boys. Of course, these were not the same men that abused him but his mind recognized that if the police were arresting these men that meant they were wrong and at fault!

God, the divine intervened as I asked, pleaded and offered my soul's tears for this man's years of pain. We heal through community and divine intervention.

The avenues that this can happen are many. If we allow ourselves to recognize that we are a spark of the divine. My knowingness of this goes back to my own childhood. I just knew that God existed. My soul knew and remembered. I attended catholic school and every day at playtime I would go to the statue of mother Mary and talk with her. I felt a calmness and peace as I connected with the divine. I didn't have cognitive knowledge of this at my young age but I had

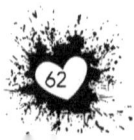

intuitive knowledge at that young age. Teaching our young ones about their emotional bodies, about their intuitive minds, that they are spirits having human experiences can help shield them from some of the human challenges they will face. Their internal strength will increase. It's similar to teaching a developing athlete how to use mental imagery and mental strength to power their athleticism.

Self-love develops as we allow ourselves to be loved. The example above illustrates how this middle-aged man allowed me to teach him self-love by providing a sacred space for him to grow and see himself, his true self. I was the mirror and I consistently reflected back to him the original love that he is. He was eventually able to forgive himself, understand his family of origin and heal his emotional human wounds. This in turn led to self-love.

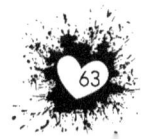

About the Author

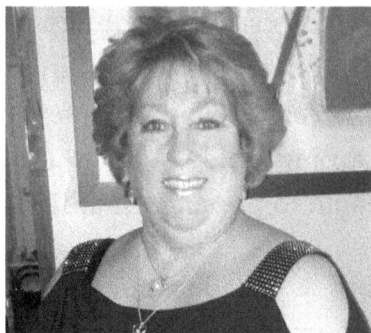

Dr. Kathleen McNulty

Dr. Kathleen McNulty studied and trained in the field of behavioral, emotional and mental health for over 35 years. She is a certified Medium, a certified Psychic, a licensed Clinical Social Worker, a licensed Marriage and Family therapist and a licensed Practicing Clinical Psychologist. As a child, Dr. Kathleen McNulty experienced paranormal phenomena. Psychic information as well as mediumistic experiences were common. As a developing young person, she became aware of the human condition, specifically curious of why humans hurt each other. Her curiosity surrounded the physical, psychological and spiritual functioning of the human organism as well as human relationships/community.

As a young adult now training in the field of psychology, Dr. McNulty was in a seminar with 24 other trainees. The presenter was a psychiatrist who was the protégée of the supervising psychologist. While listening to the presenter, Dr. McNulty became very aware that something was very wrong with the psychiatrist presenting the seminar. After the lecture she

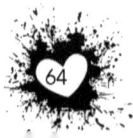

asked several of her colleagues if they were concerned for the presenter. The response was: "of course not, he is fine". Dr. McNulty dismissed her intuitive knowledge. The next morning Dr. McNulty arrived at the training facility to find many staff with their heads down and the atmosphere solemn. The presenter had taken his life the night before. That was 35 years ago. Since that time, Spirit was reawakened in Dr. Kathleen McNulty. She continued in the field of healing through the psychological therapeutic process with an in-depth understanding of how our human organism develops on this earth environment and in connection with Others. What she was always silently aware of was the presence of Spirit and the Divine working through her. Dr. McNulty quietly served all those who sought healing. She also researched the intersection of spirituality and the psychological process of healing. Dr. McNulty sought out a teacher/mentor who could further train and disseminate deeper understanding of the Spirit realm and how the Divine works through us. Dr. Kathleen McNulty was led to James Van Praagh. James Van Praagh has provided the invaluable teachings and experiential/ practice learning through his school: JVP School of Mystical Arts. Dr. Kathleen McNulty practices mediumship and psychic readings for those seeking to connect with their loved ones who have passed over. Soul to Soul communication, blending with Spirit has always been present. Spirit has guided her life since childhood. Dr. Kathleen McNulty's practice is from the heart, connecting through love and compassion. She is honored and humbled to assist as a medium for those seeking healing by connecting with their loved ones.

Visit her website to make an appointment for a healing connection: www.drkmcnulty.com.

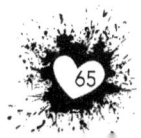

Chapter 6

Guess Who I Found Hiding Behind the Mask?

Lynn MacDonald

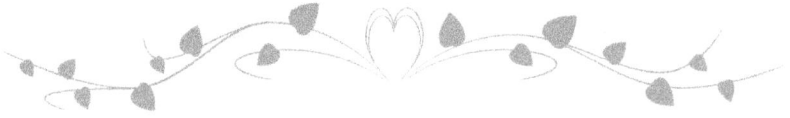

Ok, drum roll please, here's my heart-felt journey to self-love, an abbreviated version, of course! Don't worry, I won't bore you, I will only share with you all of the incredible details! I am a bit embarrassed to tell you, but while I was in the midst of "living" my life unconscious, I had absolutely no inkling that I didn't love myself. I thought I did. I never really thought about it. I had regular manicures, I had my haircut and dye jobs to cover up those greys, I was way too young to look old. I practiced self-care with a few doses of guilt.

How I woke up? I spent many years in the fitness business as I was getting older. About the time I was 46 years old, I

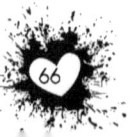

enrolled into a year-long (one weekend per month) yoga teacher training program. I thought, how hard could this be to teach? I was a physical person, I loved exercise, I just needed to prepare my body for a gentler type of modality to teach as I was getting older. We were required to meditate during the training. Mediation was foreign to me.

The first day, though I was in great shape, my body hurt sitting with a tall spine on a mat. I didn't' feel relaxed, my body held onto tension. I was annoyed and not really into meditation at all. I've never experienced stillness in my mind or body, so I was impatient, I couldn't wait for the meditations to end. My mind was busy planning, calculating, running my grocery list, thinking about the laundry, thinking about how many classes I was subbing for the upcoming week, etc. As yoga training continued, within a few months the meditations grew longer and my mind and body began to settle into the practice. I still thought about all kinds of things, my body at times still wanted to get up and move, but I was able to allow myself to surrender. I trained my mind and body to just be. An absolute miracle! Who knew?

As the months continued, I began to become more and more conscious, more aware of my life. It's like someone turned on a switch. I became aware of the disempowering words I was using to speak to myself. My self-talk was negative and extremely critical. I just never seem to find that place where I felt good enough. I became more aware of how I was feeling while interacting with certain people in my life. More aware of their negative energy. More aware than

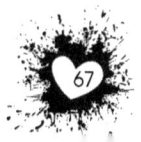

ever of what I was accepting into my life. I realized I had absolutely no standards. Well, I guess I had standards, but they were apparently way too low. I was more aware of how I was living my life or I should say really not living my life to the fullest. The more conscious I became, I realized I had absolutely no clue who the hell I was! Now, that scared me! Everything I thought was right, seemed so wrong and it felt so wrong!

Early childhood experiences often times discourage children from sharing their feelings. Lacking the ability to feel and process emotions. These early years are extremely impressive, especially when parents, family, teachers and caregivers are critical, judgmental and compare. This promotes a false sense of not feeling good enough. Living a life from the "not good enough belief system" is dangerous. We settle in life. We don't believe we could live our dreams, we don't share our gifts and talents or believe we can make an awesome living doing what we love to do. Life goes by and we run our lives off other people's belief system. I fitted very well into that category. It causes doubt, fear and it's a place where dreams never come true! A very boring non-productive and non-fulfilling place to live!

After digging deep into my soul, I developed an exercise I want to share with you. Let's get curious here for a moment. I'll ask you to grab a pen and piece of paper. Find a quite space where you can be alone and Invite into your body a few long, slow, deep relaxing breaths and just be present. Now, say out loud, "I love myself", pause and then say it

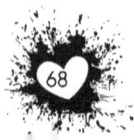

again, "I love myself", pause and one more time, "I love myself". Notice how your body <u>feels</u> as you repeat those words and contemplate the following:

1. On a scale from 0 to 100% (100% being the most) what percentage do you love yourself? Don't think about it or analyze it, just jot down the percentage, whatever comes to mind.
2. If you love yourself at 60% as an example, I want you to write out what makes up the remaining 40% that you don't love yourself. Write the words, phrases, thoughts and stories, whatever comes to mind, try not think, just allow yourself to go with the flow.
3. Notice, how you feel as you write them all out. When you are finished, re-read what you wrote. Ask yourself, how does this feel in my body? Do I believe what I wrote? Where did these beliefs come from? Are these thoughts and words my truth? What has these words and beliefs cost me in my life?

This exercise will offer new insights and help uncover specific beliefs you may have not noticed beforehand.

Luckily for my surprise "awakening", thank-you yoga! As my level of consciousness expanded more and more, my body was soaking up potent levels of self-love that was being absorbed into my tissues, cells and organs. Wow, were they dehydrated! To protect my organs, body and myself I naturally began to do the following:

• I set healthy boundaries with family and friends

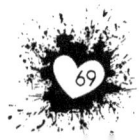

- I removed myself from people in my life whom I no longer resonated with, the ones that were incompatible to whom I was becoming
- I stopped saying yes when I meant no
- I stopped complaining, gossiping and talking about people
- I buried myself in tons of self-help books, absorbing knowledge
- I participated in several self-reflection retreats
- I spent more time alone
- I stopped watching TV, especially the news
- I began to listen to my inner voice, the one I ignored most my life
- I began to question my thoughts and beliefs. Were they mine? Did they come from other people?

As my standards and awareness began to soar to new heights, that old worn out mask I was hiding behind began to fade, shedding layers upon layers, services no longer needed, thank you very much!

I reshaped my beliefs, thoughts, feelings and emotions. This happened under the radar as part of the natural course to my journey to self-love. I just knew, as I began to make changes in my life, they felt real, they felt right! A bonus find, don't you just love when that happens? When I found what was missing, self -love, I found my self-worth, self-esteem, self-respect and self-confidence! A package-deal! They innately go together which leads of course, to yet another incredible find, introducing your true-self! No wonder why that mask I was wearing was so heavy! Your true self, a beautiful place to

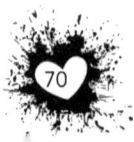

live. It's home to only you, it's real, its non-GMO, it's organic and no one else can live there!

Of course, once I found my self-love and all the other incredible surprises, my old life no longer resonated with me, I couldn't go back. I no longer fit into my old life. The rooms were full and there was no vacancy! The cost of being reunited with my self-love came with many great challenges. My changes came with hurts, fears and tough decision making which all required stepping into the realms of unknown territory. Once I got to the other side, there was a beautiful lush green path awaiting my arrival! It actually had my name on it!

I wish I met someone like myself years ago, someone who could provide me insight on self-love. I know, life doesn't come with a handbook, but certainly a self-love handbook would have helped. Then again, everyone's adventurous journey to self-love is unique and specific to them. It adds character. I felt like once I found my self-love, I naturally began to live life as the best version of myself. What a gift! I no longer took responsibility feeling like I had to people please and or make people happy. True freedom, what took so long? The best part, that old heavy ugly mask I hid behind was gone. Now, it was just me being me, real, authentic and natural.

From my heart to your heart, I would like to offer you a fresh view looking through a new set of lenses as you contemplate and tap into the wisdom of your heart to help you on your journey.

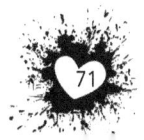

1. What would you no longer accept in your life if you loved yourself at 100%?
2. What words or phrases are part of your daily vocabulary?
3. What type of relationships do you have with yourself?
4. Does your life feel good in your body?
5. What top three emotional states do you live in on a weekly basis?
6. Is your heart open to self-love?
7. Do you know someone in your life who emulates self-love? How do they live their life? How do they talk to themselves? Do they have boundaries? Are they in loving relationships?
8. What would your life look and feel like on 100% self-love? How will you live your life? What choices would you make? What words would you speak?

Ultimately, the journey to self-love and your true self leads you to a new path that magically seems to appear. There is a beautiful path that awaits your arrival. It has your name on it! It's authentic, real with warmth and tons of sparkle and shine. It's better than you could have ever imagined!

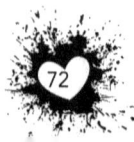

About the Author

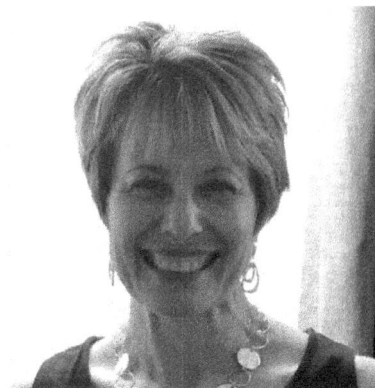

Lynn MacDonald

To learn more about Lynn, you can check out her bio and website:

https://www.spiritualguidancetoweightloss.com/

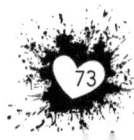

Chapter 7

How to Clear Psychic Attacks and Open Fresh to Loving Yourself

Dipal Shah

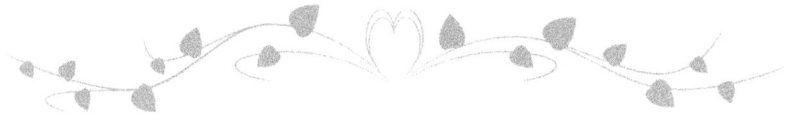

Is it their Voice or Yours?

Have you ever wondered if there is someone playing with your psyche? Have you ever considered you may be experiencing psychic attacks that can leave you feeling worthless, hopeless, physically and emotionally drained?

More and more people on the planet are having a difficult time surviving and staying balanced and centered. The energies in the environment affect every part of human existence. The universe is a macrocosm of energies. Even

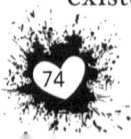

the supernatural energies ranging from angels, archangels, guides, spirits, ghosts, to the darkest of energies affect mankind. In this chapter, we are going to focus on Psychic Attacks that come from dark energies. Dark energies have various names. You may know them as entities, the devil, satan, negative thought forms, ghosts, spirits, black magic, curses, and hexes. These energies create fear, havoc and lack of self-care and love because they can take control of your body, mind and soul.

When someone is being attacked psychically, they are being controlled by a dark energy or force. They are similar to what you see in movies such as *The Exorcist* or *Poltergeist* without all of the special effects. Many people are oblivious as to how these energies even exist. Everyone at one point in their life has been exposed to a psychic attack whether or not they know or understand it. Think about a time you felt like there was someone watching you, but you turn around and no one is there or, perhaps, you felt like you heard your name, yet no one said anything.

I want you to think about these questions and write down your answer. Have you ever had an experience where you did something, but you do not recall doing it? Have you ever experienced seeing something flash by, but you look again, and nothing is there? Have you ever tried to sell your home and are doing everything right, but it just won't sell? Are any of your family members experiencing sickness again and again but there is no known medical reason for it?

If you answered yes to these questions, you may be experiencing a psychic attack.

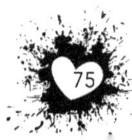

The psychic attacks I see most commonly in my practice are entities, curses, black magic, and implants. I have had the opportunity to work with thousands of people who have been through some form of psychic attack. Helping them clear these dark energies have made a profound difference in all areas of their life.

Many people think psychic attack don't exist, because they have never experienced it or paid it any attention and so they are, therefore, not affected by it. More than likely, they don't see the full picture or even the possibility that they have been attacked psychically.

I had a very special client that was very sensitive to all kinds of energy around her. She was clairvoyant, clairaudient, claircognizant, and clairsentient since she was young. She had all these abilities of awareness within her but didn't see that she had picked up a dark energy. Most of her life she dealt with health concerns, fatigue, depression, and anxiety. Doctors could not help her. When I questioned her if she ever played with the Ouija Board she said "Yes, I have." Once this energy was cleared, her health started to normalize and most of the symptoms started to disappear.

As another example, I had a client who was trying to sell her home and it would not sell no matter what she did. She was trying to move out as quick as possible and did not want to pay two mortgages. There were many homes she loved that came and went but she was unable to buy because she hadn't sold her home. She had no idea that the reason could be

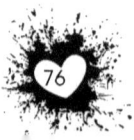

spiritual until I explained to her about the entities (a form of psychic attack) that were on her property and affecting her home. She finally allowed me to clear the psychic attack and her house sold within 2 weeks. Psychic attacks are real, and they can influence many areas of your life.

From newborns to adults, everyone attracts all kinds of energy because we are energy. Scientists have proven this through the study of Quantum Physics that everything is made up of energy. It has also been discovered that we attract energy within our subconscious minds. Some of the energies we attract are good and some are not so good. This can be scary for many. I want to help you to be aware of what to look out for before you run to the doctor or think you are going crazy. Because of your previous lack of awareness of this subject, you may have thought that things that happen within your body, relationships or even finances has to do with you all the time. Some of it certainly does, but not all of it. Sometimes whatever you are seeing, or feeling may not be a result of you or your actions. For example, have you ever been to the doctor and he/she says, "We can't find anything wrong" or "We don't know what it is, and we are doing all the tests"? If your doctor cannot give you an answer, you may want to consider asking yourself "Have I been psychically attacked?"

The most common types of psychic energies I encounter with clients are entities, curses, implants and black magic. Let me explain each in detail.

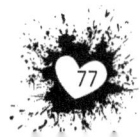

Entities

Entities are dark beings that exist on a level of consciousness where shapes aren't as fixed as they are in the physical. They attach to people and gather as much energy as they can from their host in order to survive. They are mischievous in nature, hard to control and even harder to get rid of. They attach to humans to control their behavior. Entities do not care about boundaries and believe it is perfectly okay to come into our energy field.

The person who is being attacked by an entity assumes they are responsible for creating the ongoing patterns of negative thoughts and undesired emotional responses they are experiencing. Therefore, they end up owning the entity's energy as their own. These people eventually believe that this is who they are. They live out their lives surrounded by these misconceptions and feel powerless to change.

A few weeks ago, I had a session with a client who knew something was just not right in her home. She had moved to this new home about 5 years ago and her husband loved buying antiques. He furnished and cluttered up the entire home with antique furniture. Ever since they had moved into the home, she had been unwell. She was constantly having migraines and unexplained mood swings. As I was working with her, I could see the entities were seeping in from the antiques her husband bought and causing problems within her.

On a more personal note, I will never forget the time when my daughter, who was 7 years old, told me about an entity

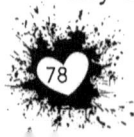

who kept harassing her and wanted her soul. I didn't know much at the time about how to get rid of this kind of psychic attack and tried to give her advice to be strong. I could see she was starting to lose herself over time. She would not sleep because she knew he would come. One day she said to me "Mom, he said he wants my soul." As you can imagine, that totally freaked me out. As a mom and energy healer new to this type of information at the time, I did my best to guide her as she is a very sensitive soul. I have had to teach her how to protect herself from these kinds of energies. About 2 years later, she was having really bad dizzy spells. Coincidentally, I had just learned how to clear entities, so I talked with my daughter's body asking it what was causing these dizzy spells? I was told clair-audiently that it was fear and I asked further what is the fear about? I was told an entity. Later that day, I asked her to tell me what she was so scared of and she told me about these spirit girls that come visit her every time she gets in trouble and they make fun of her. I had no idea this was even happening. Then she mentioned the man who wanted her soul. She said, "he is back." I was so fired up at this point that I immediately took her to my healing room and cleared 8 entities including "the man." I was shocked and exhausted at the time. After that she never had dizzy spells again!

Curses

Curses are not a thing of the past, they still exist to present day and affect modern day life. A curse is a specific intention that is imposed upon you for your misfortune by someone

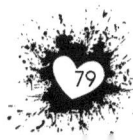

else. There are many forms of curses such as the evil eye, spells, hexes, voodoo, as well as verbal and written curses.

Curses can cause loss of finances, material possessions or opportunities. Additionally, they can cause feelings of anxiety, being "stuck" in life, illness or even death to you or, worse yet, your whole family as curses can be passed down through ancestry. As with most psychic attacks, most people who have been cursed are not aware of it. A few ways to tell are if it suddenly seems like everything is going wrong in your life, if your plants die all of a sudden or your pet isn't acting like themselves and gets sick without warning.

About a month ago, I worked with a client who had a terrible relationship with her mother. She couldn't understand why her love wasn't enough. She suffered through various ailments leaving her with adrenal fatigue and circulation issues in her body. She could sense that something was not right but didn't know what. I was able to discover that she had been cursed and got the curse to reveal itself so I could remove it. It turns out that the curse was put within this young woman when she was in womb and affected her relationship with her mother her whole life until I was able to help her.

Implants

Implants are within someone as a result of their past or present life. They act exactly like they sound, similar to a medical device that has been implanted. Implants act like a curse but are more concentrated within the body

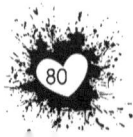

or energy field. Implants come from one's belief system and create negative thought forms about the self. Implants can also be integrated within any part of the body creating genetic disease or ailment. In my practice, I see them most commonly in the body such as the brain or organs.

Implants are like a computerized chip that has been in place for many lifetimes and placed in your present time since you were conceived. Implants are energies that are within your body or mind that have passed either from birth or at a very early age.

I recently worked with a client who wanted to enhance her spiritual gifts and had no idea what was blocking her. As we started to dive deeper into what had been the root cause of this blockage, I removed an implant within an organ in her body that was hindering her ability to grow spiritually. Immediately she could feel the tingling within her whole body and her hands.

Black Magic

Black Magic is similar to a curse, but a more potent form of dark energy used mostly by pagans, witches and practitioners of the dark arts via supernatural powers or magic for evil and selfish purposes. Black magic is malicious and can cause harm, misfortune, destruction when used for personal gain.

For example, I worked with a client who could not get out of a divorce. She was so upset because her husband wanted

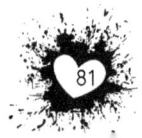

to take her child away from her to punish her and leave her empty. She had no home, no food, and no money. After many long and exhausting court battles, she had come to me for help. We found out that her husband's mother was casting a spell on him that was making him act this way. Once that was removed, she found a home and a job to support her and her daughter and her ex-husband stopped.

I worked with a young lady, 42 years of age who was abused as a child, abandoned by her father, and her mother was a narcissist. As a child she raised herself and her 2 siblings. This young lady was a very sensitive soul (one who senses energy easily). She was not married and lived a lonely life. As she was driving one day and got into an accident. She couldn't remember what had happened or how it happened. She ended up in the hospital with a broken pelvis, ribs, and many bruises. A few months later she got into another accident. Before she really realized it, she had been in 11 accidents and by now she had reconstructive surgery to her face due to all the accidents and still managed to survive. This is when she got addicted to narcotics and wanted to get off of them but couldn't. She scheduled a session with me, and we managed to clear and release implants, spirits and entities that were attached to her body, in her energy field and even some that were attacking her from a distance. She finally felt in her body and no longer on any medication.

Here is a list of how psychic attacks can be affecting YOU?

- You may experience having nightmares or frightening and unpleasant dreams.

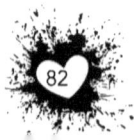

- You may see your attacker in a devilish way and dreams.
- You may be experiencing fatigue and feeling tired and depleted of energy constantly, for no reason.
- You may be feeling pain or having aches in the same place and time on a regular basis.
- You may be feeling weakness or experiencing illness or pains in areas of weakness that the attacker is aware of.
- You may be experiencing a lack of concentration and laziness regarding daily tasks.
- You may start having severe headaches or having unusually painful headaches accompanied by vomiting or dizziness.
- You may be feeling indecisive and doubtful. Questioning or doubting direction in life, even after having been aware of direction beforehand.
- You may be sensing that you are being watched.
- You may be feeling suicidal.
- You may be feeling like you are having a heart attack.
- You have lost all joy in your life.
- Your business is not making money.
- You can't find love.
- You are self-sabotaging your progress consistently.
- You have persistent health, financial, and other setbacks.
- You are hearing voices or an inner voice that constantly criticizes you.
- You have repeating patterns of behaviors.
- You are having anxiety or panic attacks.

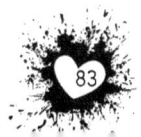

- You have irrational bouts of fear, anger, sadness or guilt.
- You have sudden changes in behavior or mood swings.
- You have addictive behaviors, including addiction to alcohol, drugs, cigarettes, sex or gambling.
- You have illnesses that will not respond to treatment or are of an unknown cause.

Granted, everyone can have a bad day. However, it has been my observation that if any of these issues are persistent in your life, then it may be a good idea to find out if you are being attacked psychically.

If you think you are being psychically attached, start to pay attention to your aura/energy field. Notice if you feel some heat or tingling in and around your body. Perhaps you notice it in one location verses all over your body? Do you feel as if someone is standing extremely close to you or watching you? These are all indications that somebody or something is in your personal space.

Psychic attacks can affect many parts of our lives including our body, mind and spirit.

When you start thinking less of yourself, judging yourself, criticizing yourself, and having suicidal thoughts you are most likely under a psychic attack.

Psychic attacks can cause a lot of interferences and so called "setbacks," most unknowingly mainly due to our differences in vibrations. The feelings of worthlessness,

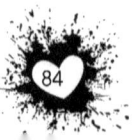

shame, abandonment, and maybe even guilt may start to creep up even stronger. Your childhood trauma may start to come to the surface more and give you setbacks as you go through life's processes. You may find you lack motivation, suffer from brain fog, as well as feel depressed, disengaged with others, angry, moody and self-absorbed.

Psychic attacks can block your growth in in your career, relationships, self-image, self-worth, spiritual growth, and mind. These energies penetrate through the energy field /auric field when we are most vulnerable. We are high vibrational beings, or we can be if we choose to be. Many times, I see people with some form of addiction, drug abuse, depression, anxiety, and they are most vulnerable to psychic attacks. I'm not saying one drink and you will attract these energies, but these energies are waiting for you to start drinking so that they can feed off you and live through you. It's like a bug. If you have ever seen the movie *Venom*, where the slimy parasite enters the body and then controls it, it is like that.

When someone is under psychic attack, most people can't think straight or function. You may feel like you aren't in your body. You stay in pain, have scary dreams, can't sleep at night, hallucinate, feel like someone is watching you, feel like you are being controlled, don't know who you are anymore, feel depressed, sad, or angry all the time.

I had a client who had so much anxiety that she could not get off the high doses of anxiety medication she was on. She would shake in her body every day. She could not get

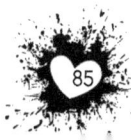

past the fear and worry she was holding onto in her life. She asked me to help her overcome this anxiety she had since she was a young girl. We had found a curse that her mother had instilled within her since birth that was causing all these issues.

How do these psychic attacks enter?

There are many different biofields that regulate various mental, emotional, spiritual, or physical functions and these correspond to various parts of the body. Scientists have been investigating the existence of these energy bodies or fields. A field consists of bands of energy called the energy field or auric field connecting the person to the outside world.

Psychic attacks may enter through the energy field or through the chakras. They may stay within the energy field and control the person from outside the body. Chakras are a system of energy vortexes along your spine. There are 7 chakras and the psychic attacks enter specifically through the 1st, 3rd and 7th. When psychic attacks enter through the chakras, they can attach to any part within the body causing disease, distress, or discomfort.

Did you ever think you needed protection? *Well You Do*

The reason you need to protect yourself from psychic attacks is because they can have an impact in every part of your life. I have had so many clients come to me because they know they are being awakened in the middle of the night by something and they are not sure what it is and

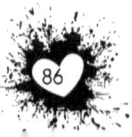

now they cannot sleep which leads to exhaustion and lack of focus. I have had clients that have psychic attacks within the thyroid and now there is a malfunction of the thyroid gland. Psychic attacks not only affect health but also career, finances, finding a home, feeling safe in your home, feeling safe in your body, your property, your car, your family. Therefore, you need protection each and every day.

Here are ways to protect you and your loved ones from psychic attacks

- Clearing Ceremony – Every culture or religion practice some form of cleansing ceremony for their homes or bodies. You can use white sage or incense. Incense such as Palo Santo helps to keep negative energies at bay.
- Use a Crystal – One of my favorite crystals is Black Tourmaline. It is a great stone to keep in your pocket, backpack, purse, wallet, and in different areas of your home. If you or someone you know is experiencing nightmares try using a Black Tourmaline. It doesn't' have to be a big stone.
- Ask the Entities to Leave – Many people do not practice the word "NO" and "LEAVE." If you feel like you are under psychic attack, tell the energy to leave. Imagine this energy leaving whichever area of your life you see it affecting. And then see your life the way you want it.
- Cut Cords – This is something that is very crucial. You create a thread of energy between you and others. You take on their energies. You can exchange psychic

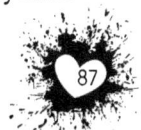

attacks as well. It is very important to clear cords from these people that you have been involved with. You can do this by asking Archangel Michael to cut cords as you take your right hand, lift it up to the top of your head and swoop it down along your spine down to your hips. Do this three times. Repeat this affirmation as you cut the cord with the swoop of your hand "I release energetic attachments so that I may serve my higher purpose." You can practice this before you go to bed each night.

- Imagine a Golden Light – You want to imagine a golden light around you to strengthen your energy field each morning before you leave your home. Imagine this light illuminating around your and protecting you from all negative energies.

- Self-Care – Many times psychic attacks occur due to lack of self-care. When you are at your most vulnerable state of mind, that is when psychic attacks occur. The best way to self-care is by taking the time to breath. Get fresh air, eat foods that are healthy for you, ground your energies by connecting to the earth, live your life consciously, meditate, and journal. This will help clear out unconscious thought patterns that do not serve you and bring you to a state of more peace and love for yourself.

Hopefully, with this information, you will be more self-aware of psychic attacks and how you can protect yourself as well as your loved ones from their harmful effects on your lives.

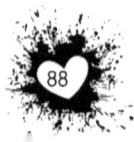

About the Author

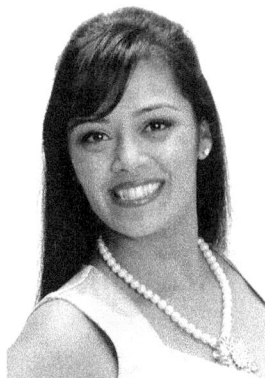

Dipal Shah B.S., MBA

International Speaker, Master Healer, and Teacher

From a pharmaceutical, biochemistry, and business background, I have transformed my life from an often stressful career on a path that brought me to an awakened spiritual journey of healing. As part of my journey, I have learned not only to heal myself and my family, but to bring awakening and healing energy to thousands of clients throughout the world.

As an International Speaker, Medical Intuit, Transformational Teacher and Master Healer, I have the ability to assist my clients in shifting their consciousness and perception in the areas of their life that are needed from relationships, health, abundance and much more. All my clients have their unique situation and my job is to guide that through energy healing.

I have helped many people of all ages including Medical Practicioners, Lawyers, Business men and women, Hollywood stars, Healers, and Alternative Healing Practicioners and young infants and children. My work has also helped pets. After

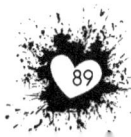

studying multiple modalities, I have developed Quantum Body Awakening as a specific type of healing. An energetic technique for healing that balances every organ, gland, and system in the body. I combine Energetic and Medical knowledge that bridge the vastness of each area. I will guide you to connect to your body as a whole and address any mis-alignments along the spine. I will dive within your body to release and dissipate any emotional and physical blockages.

My mission is to help you release the pain, illness, and dis-ease that hold you back from discovering and achieving your true purpose in life. Quantum BBodyAwakening brings instant release of balance to my clients, as this is truly my specialty.

www.Ananda4Life.com

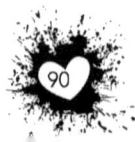

Chapter 8

My Summer of Mani-love

Gayle Nicholson

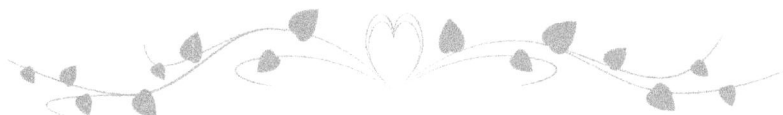

I've been a fan of Barry Manilow's music for more than four decades. It has played a significant part in my recovery from Adverse Childhood Experiences

I sat across from Alex on her couch. It was the Tuesday after Memorial Day and I was gushing about my adventures the prior weekend in Las Vegas. My hands gestured like hummingbirds in flight, flitting and zipping around in my excitement while I gave her the highlights.

"I'm going back for his birthday weekend," I finished. "Fans from all over the country, probably some from Great Britain, too, and I think one of the girls from Japan will be coming to celebrate with us in Vegas. My friends from Chicago and Detroit asked me to come party with them."

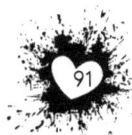

"Have you ever met him?" she asked.

"Once," my excitement settled a bit. "I waited in line for two hours in a winter coat with a two-year-old in tow to meet him at a record signing. When I finally got to the front of the line, I was so overwhelmed I couldn't form words. I felt like he must think I'm an idiot to have named my daughter, Mandy. It was embarrassing." My hands came to rest in my lap and I looked at my rings. On my left hand, a diamond engagement ring in a Tiffany setting, slim and warm glowed from my third finger. On my right, a carat of baguettes and marquis cut diamonds formed a crown of protection around a 1.75 carat solitaire. It was flashy, classy and even though it was my wedding ring from my previous marriage, I had paid for it and I felt I had "earned" the right to continue to wear it as my right-hand diamond. A daily reminder that I am *not* the marrying kind.

"He does offer a Platinum, though," I mused a bit.

"What's that?" Alex prompted.

"It's an opportunity to meet with him for 10 minutes or so if you donate a certain amount to his charity. It's *really* expensive. Last I heard, the minimum contribution was over two grand, but you get a front row seat and champagne and I hear they treat you really well, sending you home with pictures and everything."

"Have you ever done it? Platinum?"

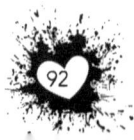

"Oh no! No way. Are you kidding? I couldn't spend that much just to embarrass myself. Not a chance. I couldn't even speak last time. Besides, what would I say?"

And then I stopped. "No, that was a lie." I marveled at my own ability to call myself out. "That's not true. I know myself as someone who can say anything, and clean it up if I need to, no problem. It's not that I'm afraid I'm going to make a fool of myself."

Alex's tattooed-on eyebrows arched. "Truth. What is it?"

"It's that I'm just *unwilling* to spend that much money on myself." The truth popped out of my mouth and left it open in amazement.

"So, you're going to do it?" Alex prodded.

"No," my eyes went wide, just the thought of it shocked me. I couldn't make that sort of jump that fast, it was too abrupt. "But I can choose to be *willing*," I said, choosing it as I spoke. "I wonder what's possible now?"

❖ ❖ ❖

Two weeks later I got a message from an old fan club friend. She'd scheduled a Platinum package and now, unfortunately, her mother's health was failing, and she didn't feel good about leaving town. The Platinum packages were non-refundable. If she didn't find a person to take over her package, she would lose everything she paid for it.

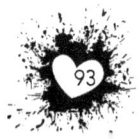

Coincidentally, (...hahhahhah, you know better than that, dear reader) I'd recently received money that would pay for my return trip to Las Vegas to celebrate Barry's birthday weekend with my friends from the Midwest, plus a little extra. I offered her as much as I could, knowing I'd still have to afford a room and food for the Platinum date in late July.

But this was just the beginning. With my new-found willingness to spend money on myself for the sake of my own joy and full self-expression, I visited Las Vegas 6 times between Memorial Day and Thanksgiving. I was able to see his show 12 times in total. It never got old. I can hardly describe the up-levelling I experienced, mentally and emotionally, not to mention financially, over those few short months that went by so very fast.

A few experiences stuck in my mind. The highlights, if you will, that became the memories to last a lifetime. For example, the conversation during my platinum visit where I almost made Barry feel bad for cancelling the shows on his birthday weekend, but I think in the end I made him see it was all ok. That was awkward.

Then there was the "slightly inappropriate question" I asked him that got me a true smile in our "official portrait". He laughed, chuckled, actually. It was music to my ears. Kirsten, Barry's tribe member that escorted each of us into the meeting room, said, "That's one for the books," as she escorted me out, chuckling a little herself. I blogged about it here. (https://misfitsandmiracles.com/).

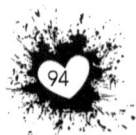

I'm not going to lie, there were a few times that my breath hitched in my chest and I felt my spine stiffen. How was I going to cover all of this? And then the money just showed up. It was like nothing I had ever seen before. During one of my visits, I won enough to cover the next, and so on. I went in May, June and July, but in August Barry was in the UK for a month and I stayed home. In September, he was back and I celebrated my own 50th birthday with a weekend of champagne and self-indulgence. Even though I went back again in October for the cancelled birthday make up shows, and in November "just because" I wanted to see a couple Manilow friends while they were in town for the shows. It was glorious letting myself say yes, trusting that whatever happened, everything was gonna be all right.

It was my birthday weekend that I bought the star necklace. I'd wished for it for years, but it seemed a little pricy. Almost a hundred dollars for a gold-plated replica that resembled what he wore on the cover of his Greatest Hits album. Nevertheless, in the interest of celebrating my achievement of surviving for half a century, I decided to splurge and bought it. The plating on the side that touched my chest began wearing thin within a couple of days, so I returned to the shop and exchanged it.

The necklace that adorns my neck today is the exact copy of the necklace from the album cover. White gold, with a genuine diamond sparkling from the center. It's my talisman now. My good luck charm. It is my star that reminds me to believe in myself.

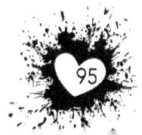

I imbued it with the power to remind me that I can achieve anything with courage and consistency. I already have. Now is the time to share my experience, strength and hope with you.

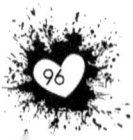

About the Author

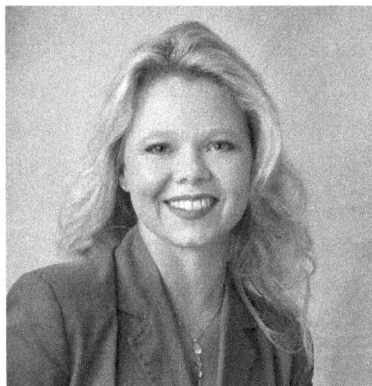

Gayle Nicholson

A survivor of childhood sexual abuse, kidnapping, severe neglect, and the psychological trauma of being abandoned multiple times, Gayle developed a certain skill in overcoming horrific life experiences. Drawing from her experiences as a survivor of adverse childhood experiences she shares her wisdom in the hope that people who have experienced early trauma like hers will be helped by it.

Gayle holds degrees in Journalism and Metaphysical Science and has a lifetime of experience in pushing past normal into extraordinary. Through the many self-help and personal development programs she's studied, she developed a unique ability to listen to a person's tone and word choice to intuitively hone in on the core of an issue, allowing her to get to the root of a problem quickly and clear it efficiently. Best of all, she shares her experience in such a way that you will find it easy to apply her empowering techniques to your own life to produce extraordinary results today, tomorrow, and every day to come.

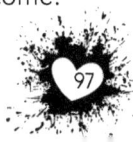

If you are an Entrepreneur woman who has suffered 4 or more of the 10 Adverse Childhood Experiences identified by the Kaiser-Permanente ACE Study (https://en.wikipedia.org/wiki/Adverse_Childhood_Experiences_Study), Gayle offers a program that can help release you from the unproductive cycle of recreating patterns from the past. The 40 Day Reset addresses the top five areas of life where adverse childhood experiences are most likely to have created barriers in your brain, clearing them in a way that traditional talk therapy never will. Visit www.GayleNicholson.com for more information today. You've suffered enough.

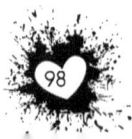

Chapter 8

Joyful Attitude

Leonora Castillo

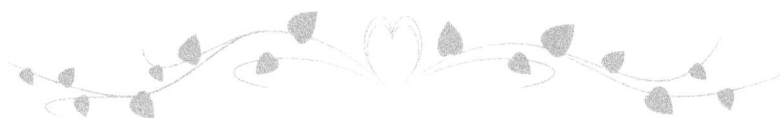

When you get to the end of everything you know,
Know that there is something to stand on, or
You will be given wings to fly.
~ anonymous

Learning to love myself is number one on my list to show myself that this is the care I need. As women, we tend to care for everybody in our family first, and then we take care of ourselves. I learned that, just like "the talk" on the planes about getting the oxygen mask, yes, we all know that one. Put the mask over your face first, and then put it on your young child. I need to take care of myself first, so I can take care of others. Others for me now, include my family, of course, and my friends, and the people who have no voice – to stand in the gap for them, so I can speak for them.

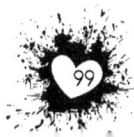

Loving myself, doesn't mean material things. One thing that I fight myself about, is judgement. When I retired from corporate world, which is so very recent, about 2 months, I began to write an online course about charity giving and how it is good for companies to have a giving plan. This is all new to me. I have done a lot of research, while I am running our own charity. My internal conversations sometime lead me to: Who am I to do this? What right do I have to tell other people what to do? There are more qualified. I don't know what I'm doing. These are internal conflicts and judgement that I must overcome each day. I just know, because I have a passion about helping people, that I will succeed. My daily affirmations help me. I keep a journal, where every day I write 10 things that I am, and 10 things that I'm grateful for. I listen to praise and worship music, study the bible, listen to my mentor online, and pray. This is what I do, before I start my day. It sets up my day to be joyful, have a great attitude, to be kind to others, to negate all the negative thoughts. I call this -primed.

The most important thing you can do to love yourself is to give yourself permission to explore new things. Explore your unique gifts and talents. I have committed to as lifetime of learning. The only way you can explore and find out more about your gifts is to pray hard and see what's out there. Be curious. Also, see who is out there. Get out of your circle and go to conferences where you might meet people who like the same things and think like you do. If what they are doing interest you, keep up with that relationship and get to know them better. It might open doors and opportunities for you that you never thought possible. The funny thing

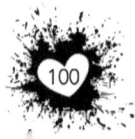

about exploring, is that you find out that there are so many things that exist that you had no idea about. With all the new technologies sprouting everywhere, there are millions of these. I love gardening. This is only home gardening, so I've watched a lot of videos about gardening. One of the things I found was farmers cannot plant the same crops on the same soil every year. They either must rotate their crops or let the land be empty for a time so it can replenish the minerals and other things in the soil, for a good yield next time. There was one event that my husband and I went to in Arizona, and I started talking to a gentleman, who happens to have a booth in the conference. His company use algae and inject them into the soil so that farmers will have better crops and better yield and will replenish the soil without letting it go fallow for a year or so. Wow! Something I would never think about. We are good friends now, and we keep in touch every month.

Follow up with people who interest you. This is a key ingredient in sales. If you are in sales, you have heard this so many times – The money is in the follow up. It turns out, it's not just money that's in the follow up. Relationships are built and friendships deepen in the follow up. Let's not stay so busy that we neglect calling or sending out emails to those we like and love. I know it's the new age, and not too many people send snail mail anymore. When my granddaughter, she's seven years old, got an award at school, I sent her a handwritten card through the mail, and she loved it. Occasionally, it's a good idea to just reach out and send a card.

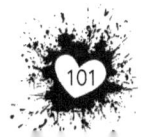

When I was 17, my family moved to the US from the Philippines. We are a family of six, mother, father, two sisters and one brother. Being born in the suburbs of Manila, means we have access to the big city and all that it entails. My father, a very courageous man, moved us all here knowing that there are no opportunities for his children where we were. At 17, I had already finished high school and one year of college at a famous technical and engineering school called Mapua Institute of Technology, in Manila. Over the years, I worked as computer chip designer at several high-tech companies in Silicon Valley. The chips, I've helped designed are widely used commercially, including home appliances, cell phones and the new driverless cars. The technology is cutting edge, submicron, nanotechnology. I started working in August 1973 and retired November 2018. I know, I know, that's a lot of years in corporate. 15 years of that, I was self-employed and did the same work in technology, but I worked as a consultant for several companies. I was raising my three kids, and being a consultant gave me more freedom with my time to spend with my family.

Since I retired, my calendar is full. Talk about busy. I am running a non-profit organization to raise money for emergency shelter for survivors of human trafficking. I am also launching a new online course to train non-profits how to qualify for more funding. Meeting people whether online meetings or physical meetings take up a lot of time. I am also, since November one of the Board Members of Silicon Valley Shakespeare. My son announced at a family gathering, "mom retired so she can work more." So true, but these are things I am passionate about.

My calendar is full, yes. Like I said, I start my day with a great attitude. I also schedule my work out time each day. I am proactive with my health. Not always, but most days I eat the right foods. There are some foods, I know shouldn't eat, but once in a great while, I will eat them. I love chips and spicy salsa and spicy guacamole. That's one thing I would let myself eat, along with chocolate. My kids, and nieces make fun of me, because, when they were growing up, I would hide my chocolates. They all pretend that they didn't know where they were, so I can have a little bit of fun. Every year, my husband and I join people all over the world who fast for 21 days at the beginning of the year. Along the way, I found out the fasting helps your body to reset. Hippocrates said, "Let food be they medicine." This year, we are doing water fast, with some pure apple juice and cranberry juice. Fasting also detoxify your body. Fasting brings a deeper connection with my God. I am waiting for some revelations that will propel my projects forward, or shut them down fast, so I don't waste my time on them,

Laughter is a good medicine. We all heard that, right? But can you also laugh at yourself? This is one of the keys to loving yourself. Don't judge yourself. Be open to laughter. Sometimes I would be walking and think of things I have done, and I would start laughing -all by myself. I don't really care who's looking at me. Ok, sometimes, I bring my phone to me ear, and pretend I'm talking to someone. I accept my faults and weaknesses. I don't worry about things that are out of my control.

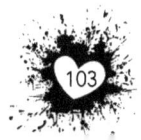

I like my workspace clean and tidy. But it usually doesn't stay that way all the time. I have my crochet project on my desk, several notebooks for my journal, hand lotion, essential oils, several colored pens and pencils, books, two kindle, one phone, several mugs and glasses. Chaos, right. There is some order to them though. When I put away dishes and groceries, I put them in the general area where I think they should be, which is where there's room in the cabinets and pantry. I always get in trouble with the kids and my husband for this. Now they just laugh along with me. Hey, if they want to put them away, go for it. I also used to pull pranks on my family, so when family camp comes along, the teenagers will approach me as soon as we get to camp and ask what we are going to do this time, or I want to be on your team.

My family camps out on 4th of July. Extended family also comes, so we can be anywhere from 40-60 people. We divide ourselves into two teams, and game on for the rest of the 4 days. Husband and wife cannot be on the same team, as well siblings. One of the things we did as prank was, scraping out the cream out of the Oreos and replace them with toothpaste. This went very well. The other one that didn't go well was, we duct tape the zippers of the tents in the wee hours of the morning. You can imagine why, that didn't go well...

If we don't laugh at ourselves, our response might be judgement. NO one can make us feel worse about ourselves than we can. We are the only ones who can give others permission to put us down. Knowing who you are, and being confident on being who you are, lets you be gentler

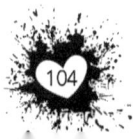

with yourself. People can say negative things about you, but you don't have to receive it. My friend Sharon Lechter said, take your right hand, brush away on your left shoulder, as if getting the lint off you. When you hear negative comments about you or was told something you don't want to receive, do that. This is your code, our code that you are brushing away negative things away from you. (Sharon Lechter is the author and co-author of the Rich Dad Poor Dad series along with Robert Kiyosaki)

Unconditional self-acceptance. What does that mean? It means, whatever I did wrong yesterday, or any other time in the past, accept it. If I did something wrong to someone, ask for forgiveness. A few years ago, I wrote a letter to each one of my three kids and ask them for forgiveness. I asked forgiveness for different things from each one of them. Don't get me wrong. My kids and I have great relationship even before those letters. They were surprised when they got them. Most importantly, forgive yourself. Believe me, it takes a lot practice, forgiving myself. When you can forgive yourself easily, know that you can also forgive others easier and faster. When you do this, you will be happier and have a better attitude every day.

Recognize my wins and celebrate them. Each day, as I finish the day, I go back to my calendar and my OneNote (this is where I categorize my to-do lists), to see what I have accomplished today, and what I put off for tomorrow. Some days are good, and some days are not so good. Keeping a journal, that I can carry around is a great way to keep the reminders going. When I write things on paper, it keeps it

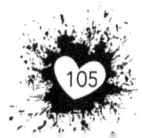

out of my head. I know when I write it down, I will see it again later as a reminder, so I don't have to carry it around in my head constantly or worry that I might forget something.

When there are wins, great or small, I give myself an Atta girl, and let my husband know. He is one of my greatest cheerleaders. We celebrate often. Most times when we come back from a conference, we share about who we met and who they are, and what they do. We even celebrate, when we meet new people and we can become great friends with them. One of these examples is when we were in New York, attending c-suites conference and Hero Club Conference. We met a gentleman whose business is bottled water. For every bottle they sold, they give one meal to a child. He invited us to help his non-profit where they pack 3000 meals every Thursday and give them to the kids at their school on Friday so the kids will have food for the weekend. We showed up and helped pack and met another family of four. We had such a great conversation that night, and this new family invited us for dinner to their home a couple of days later. These are great people who are changing the world by filling a need. We love them. Our new friend who owns the water bottle company invited us to go to with them to Belize, where they are spending New Year's week with his parents. Come on! I've never been to Belize, and it's warm there. They live on the beach and has room for us. It's cold where we were and raining. Summer weather, beach, vacation, sipping cold drinks, eating fresh fruits. Alas, we didn't go. We plan on going next year, though. These are all great wins for us. This kind of connections lead us to more and more great connections.

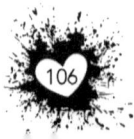

Slow down. Life won't take over. Explore new things and ideas. Meet new people. You don't know what you don't know until you get out there, way out there.

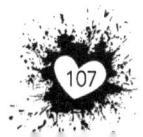

About the Author

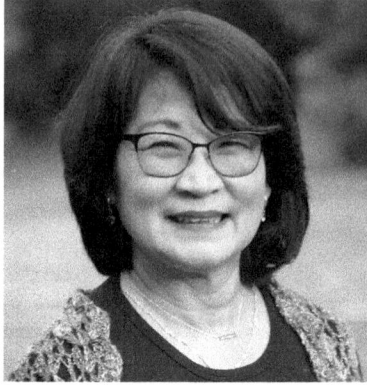

Leonora Castillo

Leonora Castillo is the co-founder of 56united, a non-profit company that raise money to provide emergency shelter to the survivors of human trafficking. Most people know about human trafficking in third world countries. They are also common in most cities of the United States. California is one of the top consumers of labor and sex trafficking. Join the movement to end slavery. Find more: www.56united360.com

Leonora also runs a company called Charity Bridge, whose purpose is to help non-profit organizations qualify for corporate funding, as well as increase their donor base to raise even more money for their programs. She trains companies that having a giving plan. A giving plan provides a great advantage for brand recognition, and customer loyalty.

She has served as a youth leader for several years at her local church, as well as serving at different local charities in the Greater Bay Area. Coming from an immigrant family, she has succeeded in carving out a career in the high-tech industry, working as a chip designer. She led a number of people in different projects and mentored them for leadership skills and lifting them up for higher consciousness of themselves as leaders and pioneers in their field.

Along with her husband, they also have a business education company to help business owners structure their companies to maximize revenues.

www.56united360.com
https://www.facebook.com/mycharitybridge/
https://www.linkedin.com/in/leonoracastillo/
https://www.facebook.com/thepathtoprofits/

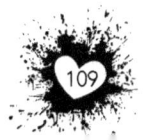

Chapter 10

Choosing You

Christine Fodor

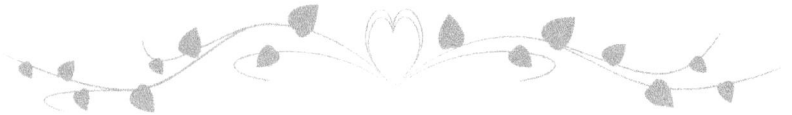

hat is not ok for you that if it was ok would set you free? Huh? Exactly! We'll come back to this question later. Everyone says you need to love yourself. Well what does that mean exactly? Sure there are times when we are critical with ourselves, judge our bodies or if this then that, like if I lose 20 more pounds then I will love myself. Ok so... we can be more gentle with ourselves, judge ourselves less, and be more kind to ourselves. That's great. And I thought I was, or at least better than I used to be. But what I found was that I didn't allow myself choice. What? Of course I had choice! Really? Do you?

So there I was at the Human Awareness Institute (HAI) workshop level 3 which is all about 'Choice'... HAI (www.hai. org) is a great organization for love, intimacy and sexuality workshops; in fact level 2 is 'Loving Yourself'. But it was level 3 'Choice' that got me. I could not choose! The exercises

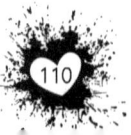

are confidential so as not to spoil the experience for others as well as honoring privacy. What I can say is that we were given different situations in which to choose and when it came time for me to choose another person for an exercise I could not choose. In fact, I almost left the building... literally! I realized that due to my spiritual beliefs and practices I let everything happen to me. I let people come to me and let others ask me or choose me and had faith that it was in divine order. And it was. It was a lesson for me to learn to choose me. It gave me an opportunity to ask myself, "If there are no rules, no reason for me to let things happen to me, what would I choose, who would I choose?" Then I realized there had always been reasons for my choices. It was never about me choosing for me for no other reason than what would I like. There always had to be calculations and explanations and who knows how many other justifications. Now all of that just seems exhausting!

For me, since I had come from a history of abuse, it had left me without boundaries and choice. The magic of that workshop was facing and speaking up about abuse and realizing choice was not safe. Huh? Yep, look at what my choices got me, an abusive marriage. Choice = pain. And if somehow I was good enough in my faith then only good things would come to me. Really? How about choosing for yourself? What you would really like to have and be? I didn't. There was always an expectation, an obligation, or what is perceived to be ok or not ok from family, society, religion. Well, what about choosing for you without any of that? That is being true to you. I thought I had free will choice. I thought I was choosing it. I wasn't. Now I know different.

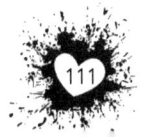

So how does choice equal self-love? Well, how much do you really choose you? Not to get a certain outcome or to avoid an outcome but real choice for the purity of what you would like? No consequences, no obligations, no shoulds, no expectations. Just you. For you. THAT'S loving you.

So what about that original question, what is not ok for you that if it was ok would set you free? It's only your perception, your point of view that makes things not ok for you. For me back then, choosing just for me was not ok. I needed a reason. And it was not ok for me to say no. Can you say no? I would worry about the other person's feelings, I thought I had to say yes to be a nice person, or it was expected. That's one of the reasons choice was so hard for me. I did not flex my muscle saying no. Another opportunity at a HAI workshop is to practice saying no and it was a bit uncomfortable but a safe place for me to build my 'no' muscle. I was always so worried, well about everything really, that I didn't want to hurt anyone's feelings or give a rejection to someone. Well what about me? I was willing to sacrifice myself, my choice, my desire to the point that I didn't even know what my choices and desires were. Is that self-love? How about self-sacrifice? And of course I had manifestation lists of things I desired to be or have but not the everyday little things moment to moment. Then I learned that it was the big things too. I was taught that choice was 'permanent' and 'suffer the consequences' of your choice. It was more like WATCH OUT for what you choose; you NEED to make the RIGHT choice. Says who? Just choose something else.

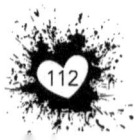

Every moment is another breath, another choice even if you choose the same thing again. If you don't like something, then choose something else. How did I get so good at choosing? I studied Access Consciousness® (founder Gary Douglas, www.accessconsciousness.com). They use choice and questions to increase possibilities which for me created freedom. And since I was already the Question Queen, I loved it! And for me, being in integrity with myself is honoring my ability to choose something else, always putting me first. That's loving me. Honoring me. Being in integrity with me. And guess what? I'm so much happier! Who says you have to suffer? F-that! Chose you and what makes you smile, makes you sing, makes you dance! Be free! Let go of obligations and expectations and what you should do because because because...

So... what is not ok for you that if it was ok would set you free? What are you not willing to choose for you that if you did would bring you more joy and more fun? Instead of weighing the consequences or if it's a right or wrong choice, just choose you. And if you're struggling with this question because of family then yes choosing them might also be choosing you and then maybe not. Only you know what that is for you. And you can change your mind at any time! That is the NOT choosing out of obligation thing. So right now maybe I am a yes and then when that day finally arrives it's a big fat no, guess what, I say no. I don't force myself to struggle through things just because I said yes. That's the honoring of you. What kind of energy do you bring when you force yourself to do something you really don't want to do? And it's not always about instant gratification. I

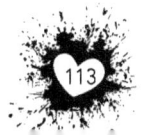

don't enjoy cleaning house but I sure do enjoy a clean house so it's worth doing. And choosing you is not being selfish. It's self-love. And I do things for others that might not be something I would choose for me by myself, but they are important to me so I choose it for them which is still for me, kinda like enjoying a clean house. And if I'm choosing everything else and I don't have a clean house that's ok too. It's all ok. It always is. You are perfect just the way you are. There's nothing wrong with you. There's nothing to fix. All you have to do is love you, choose you.

So what do you do if you don't know how to choose, or how to choose you, or there seems to be something blocking you from moving forward even though you know it will create something more for you? That's when you start to ask more questions. Would some facilitation or some energetic body work help release this energy that seems to be stuck? Choosing you sometimes means for you to ask for help or assistance to get to where you would like to go and who you would like to be. That's what I specialize in. After having been through it myself I love to help others get through it for them. See my journey to health and wellness started at age 20 with a back injury and many other injuries and ailments that followed. Now that I look back on it, most of it was when I was in that abusive marriage and didn't see a way out. It wasn't until I was driving around a curve in the country that I thought, well if I just go straight into that tree... That's when I decided to ask for help. I didn't even realize that I was ready to ask for a divorce because I didn't think divorce was a choice because of my religion. Though I realized God didn't mean for me to drive into a tree so getting a divorce would be ok. That's when I started making choices for me.

After western medicine just gave me drugs and more drugs, I finally decided to start searching. I knew there had to be something else out there. That's when I discovered alternative therapies and energy healing. It helped me! I was able to get off most of the meds. I thought to myself, people need to know about this stuff! So I began my studies and certifications to be the practitioner and facilitator I am today. And if those things hadn't happened I probably wouldn't have followed this path. I am now able to have gratitude for all of my life. Even those days that were scary at times, and there are things that I remember that were positive. It wasn't always so dark, it just got worse and it was time for me to choose. I can say that the path wasn't always easy and I had to work at it, but I never gave up. And now I'm willing to choose joy and fun and more ease. Instead of being a seeker, I became a finder. Are you willing to choose that for yourself?

When you run into roadblocks or situations that seem like there is no choice, know that you always have a choice! I chose not to drive into that tree. I chose to call someone for help. I chose to file for legal separation and get the papers served with a restraining order. I chose to leave in the middle of the night in the snow in freezing temperatures at the end of January while he was at work. I chose to call his family to be there to watch him to make sure he didn't do something crazy. All the abuse I remembered, he didn't. He was too drunk. That was 23 years ago. There's a lot more to that story but I'm sure you get where I was and see where I am now. No matter what your life is or where it's been, you can choose you at any time and you can choose to love you at any time. And at different times in your life, choosing you may look totally different. Back then it was me choosing to live a better life. And you know what? I still choose that for myself every day! Though now instead of fleeing a bad situation, it's taking a plane to go somewhere fun and experience a new adventure. What can you choose to choose you, to love you, to live a better life?

What's next? That's one of my favorite questions to ask. What is next for me? What is next for what I'm asking to create in my life? And that's actually the point... Create your life! That IS loving you. Stop being at the effect of everything and everyone around you. What would bring you joy? What would invigorate your body, your mind, your spirit? Notice the joys. The moments where your heart swells. Appreciate the little things. Celebrate the big things. And give gratitude for it all. Be grateful for all of you. All that you have been through, all that you have accomplished, and all that you have yet to be. You are a miracle. You are magic. All you have to do is choose it. What can you choose today for more self-love? And every day? And if you find it difficult or it seems like something is stopping you or blocking you, reach out to one of us who's been there and made it through. That's a loving you choice too. Be the magic miracle you be. All is available to you. If you choose it. Choose you. BE self-love.

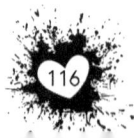

About the Author

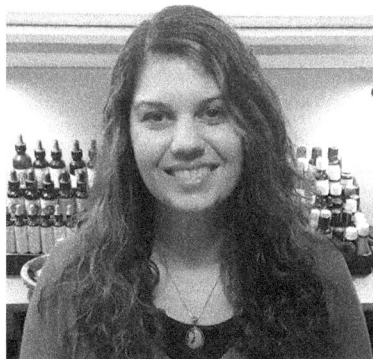

Christine Fodor

Christine Fodor is an Energy Medicine Specialist & Creation Coach specializing in working with individuals and groups to clear blocks and limitations to success in love, relationships, business, health and wealth.

Christine has been providing psychic readings and energy healing since 2003 and has been a Reiki Master since 2005. Christine has hosted her own online radio show and is an accomplished author. She teaches multiple healing modalities certification courses and has hosted many meditation and manifestation groups over the years. Christine now facilitates Creation Actualizing Events to help you bring your creations to fruition using personalized tools and techniques to bring your visions to a living reality. More information can be found at the Renewal Clearing & Healing website www.renewalhealth.net.

Christine offers in person and online healings, readings and coaching using her certifications in Access Consciousness BF,

BPF, AFF, AHP, CFMW; Certified ThetaHealer; Holy Fire III Usui and Karuna Reiki Master; Art of LIving Crazy Possible Graduate; Mahatma Initiate; Human Awareness Institute Assistant & Connect Leader; Universal Life Church Minister. Christine also has a BA from MSU in Interior Design with minors in Psychology and Communications, is a Graduated Nursing Assistant and a Licensed Physical Therapist Assistant specializing in Outpatient Orthopedics.

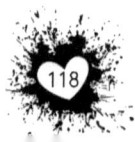

Chapter 11

Welcome to My Pity Party

Tiffany Kiefer

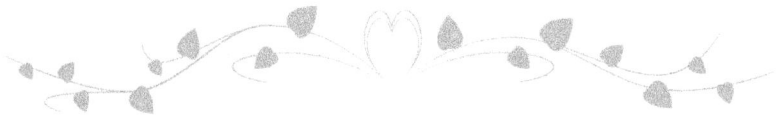

How had I gotten to such a low place in my life? Have you ever felt so humiliated that you just wanted to crawl into a hole and zip it up? I have. I was a leader and a trip earner for my direct sales company on my way to a seven-day tropical cruise that I had earned. Even though I was at the top of my game, I wanted to die. I was sitting on a plane and I was so heavy that my fat hung over into the next seat and into the isle. Yes, I always had a smile on my face, but I was so sad inside. I was a master pro at putting a "happy face sticker" on everything, but I was slowly dying inside. The flight attendant had to get me an extender to put on my seat belt in order for us to take off. I was humiliated and embarrassed, let alone uncomfortable. So was my seat mate. Every time the cart came by during our six-hour flight, it hit me. I remember thinking; just get this over with, put me out of my misery.

Then I got a wake-up call. Shortly after my daughter was born, my body stopped working from the neck down. To this day, we aren't sure what happened. I was paralyzed. I remember my husband calling 911, and when help arrived, they looked at me and couldn't figure out how to get me out of the house. It took three men to get me onto the gurney and out to the ambulance. I was humiliated. It was at that moment that I had had enough. I never, ever wanted to be embarrassed like that again. I wanted to be able to run and jump with my kids. I wanted to LIVE. I had weight loss surgery. I thought that would solve my problems. And it did, for a little while.

I was doing really well, I thought. I had gotten my weight problem under control. I became a community leader, and even a baseball coach. I felt like I had my stuff together until the morning the United States Air Force called and told us we were moving to England. My whole world was ripped out from underneath me in that very second.

I had to take my children out of school mid-year. I quit my job, stopped volunteering, left my friends, left my family and had to start completely over. You might tell yourself, this is a great thing; WOW! Living in another country, what a great experience! Well, I wasn't feeling it. You see, I went from going over 1000 miles an hour to a screeching halt. Actually, I went in reverse.

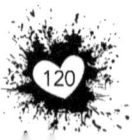

My children had instant friends at school. My husband had connections at work. I had no one. I was in a deep, deep, dark pity party all my own. I was unable to put a happy face sticker on this one. And to make matters worse, it was the worst part of winter there. It was freezing cold, snowing and DARK. I would kiss my kids goodbye every morning from my bed, and they would have to walk to school in the snow because I couldn't gather enough gumption to even get out of bed. I kept the curtains closed and the lights off and stayed in my pajamas all day. The pain I felt from missing my family was ripping my heart out every day, and not having my friends to console me was even worse. My husband didn't understand. My kids had no clue. I had no one to talk to. No one cared. I was all alone. I felt unloved, uncared for and completely lost. I was on a downward spiral, fueled by resentment, anger, loneliness and deep sadness. My own visceral HELL.

This was my life and I had to deal with it. For the next three years this was my hell... in another country, far away from anything I knew, anything I loved and anything I thought I was good at. I was here with a husband I wanted desperately to fall back in love with. I didn't even know if he wanted me. My children were struggling to find their way in a country that although beautiful, was in the dead of winter and DARK.

One morning, after I kissed my kids good bye I was lying in bed, crying, wondering "Why me?" Why was I so miserable? I was a happy person. I loved to smile. I loved helping others. What was I doing curled up in the fetal position balling my

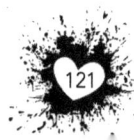

eyes out? I lay there, crying uncontrollably. You know that ugly face crying? That was me. As I paused crying for just a moment, I heard a whisper. Actually, I am lying. It was a shout. My inner voice spoke up. LOUDLY! It told me I was the problem. I was the one contributing to the HELL I was in. I was in this damaging situation because I was allowing it. As I looked around the dark room, I wasn't sure who said that. I thought "Um, who said that?" And then I heard it again... "Get UP, get dressed. It is time." Time for what I had no clue, but I did as the voice in my head said and I got up and got dressed. That day I picked my kids up at the bus stop in the car, so they didn't have to walk in the snow, the first of many days ahead of healing.

The next day I started by walking my kids to the bus stop and walking home. I began to appreciate the wonders around me. I even appreciated the different garbage cans that England had and the post office box on the corner, the local store and the beautiful flowers, the numerous gnomes in the gardens, there were many. I began to be grateful. It was then that I got a pretty journal and began to write what I was grateful for... what I appreciated about England. the simple little things. I soon made a friend and we began to get healthy together, working out twice a day, taking walks, and appreciating the simple things. I was on my way up and out of the darkness, and so was England. Spring was arriving.

It was at that time that I knew I needed to become more. I needed a purpose. But what was I good at? WOW! That is a loaded question. Really, what could I do to help with the

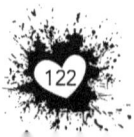

family finances? I had some business sense and I knew how to clean house, so I opened up a cleaning company. My friend advertised for me and I had my first few clients in no time. Hard work, good work ethic, and a doing a really good job, awarded me with a thriving business in England.

The more I continued to appreciate the simple things, the more BIG things came into my life. We were able to create a baseball team on the Air Force base and travel with the athletes. We enjoyed traveling to many different countries in Europe with our children. seeing sights we would have never been able to see if it weren't for me listening to that shout in my head on that dreary day. We had amazing adventures in England, learning about cultures, trying new foods, and making friends for a lifetime. When we got orders back to the USA, I sold my business to my partner, my husband Retired from the Air Force and we were starting over again, only this time we were home.

When we transitioned back to the USA, the same situation arose again, only this time I knew exactly how to handle it. I chose not to go into the fetal position. I chose to start my cleaning company at home. Actually, I was very ambitious. I started an apparel company as well to inspire others with inspirational clothing. I chose ME. I continued to be grateful every day for what God had provided my family and me. I wanted to create the reality that I can manifest anything that I truly desire. I believe that my true purpose in life is to inspire and create happiness wherever I go. I help others on their journey to be brave and manifest the life they want.

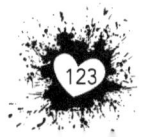

Manifestation is all about a knowing that something will happen. Believing isn't always about seeing it before it happens. It is about knowing it is going to happen and viscerally feeling the feelings of it happening and living in the moments of it happening. What do your dreams look like? What do they feel like? What does your future look like? What does it feel like? I ask myself these questions all the time. I do this in order to keep the dreams and visions alive in my heart, my head and in the universe, so that they come to fruition.

Dreaming big has always been a desire for me. But having superficial things and material goals is one thing and having spiritual goals and aspirations is completely another avenue. Being fully connected to myself is so important to me, so much more important than any material item. You cannot put a price on self-love. It is priceless. I continually touch base with my inner self to make sure that I am on the right track. I do this by meditating. I walk and meditate. That is the easiest for me. It is difficult for me to sit still for long periods of time. I am a little bit of a firecracker…hehehe. Checking in with myself keeps me grounded and helps me stay focused on the things that I want, rather than on the things I don't want.

Helping me stay focused on the things I want is being grateful for the things I have in my life. I have a beautiful gratitude journal that I write my gratitudes in daily. I tell my journal about the day that I had and the good and bad things that happened. But most importantly, I record my five gratitudes in it, five different things I am grateful for

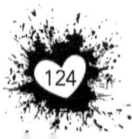

everyday, the simple ones all the way to the big ones. The more you are grateful the more wonderful things start happening in your life. Things just start to flow with ease and grace to you. It is like the universe thanking you for being thankful. It is wonderful. I even write about things in my journal that I want to happen. But I write about them as though they have already happened. Then I bask in the energy of what it feels like when they happen. I envision it happening, see it in my mind's eye, live it, play in it, and it becomes a reality. It is that simple. The true trick is to do all of this without any DOUBT!!! If you can do that, you have it made. You are a manifesting Law of Attraction expert!

Speaking of Law of Attraction, I became a Certified Coach of LOA because I wanted to help others master the powers of the universe, master how they can create their own reality and a life worth living. You may ask yourself; how do you create your reality when everyone else's reality interferes with yours. I choose not to associate with others' drama for one and for two, I focus on what I want in my life daily rather than the things I don't want. For example, when you are sick, you are constantly stating, oh my cough, oh my headache, oh my... (focusing on what you DON'T WANT) when you could focus on that fact that this is lovely. I am able to get some good rest today. I am choosing to feel good today. This tea and honey tastes so lovely. Redirecting your thoughts, however silly or crazy, gets your mind focused in a different direction, away from what you don't want, and focuses the energetic vibration in a totally different direction. Remember, "Like attracts like" or one I really like is "What I think about I bring about."

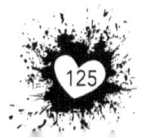

You have the choice to create your reality. YOU DO. You get to get up every single day and create the day. It is a new day every day. If you choose to continue the same shit you had yesterday, that is your choice, no one else's. Are you getting this? YOU CHOOSE. Every day I wake up and I say what I am grateful for. EVERYDAY. I do this because it puts me in a state of peace, a state of gratitude, and a state of receiving. So many times, we are constantly feeling like we have to give give give and never stop and really embrace all that we have around us, all that we are grateful for, so I do that every day. Sometimes, I do it more than just in the morning.

The more grateful I am, the more great things come to me, the more I am aligned with my inner self and my true purpose in life. I find that when I get off of this routine, everything seems to go sideways, so I have to come back to center and hone in on what I am here for and my purpose.

Create what you want. Focus on it. Look at it every day. I have a vision board. Actually, I have a few. (Guilty: I want to create a lot of things in my reality.) When you place things in your VISION on a daily basis what happens? You tend to see more of it, right? When you want to buy a particular car, you start seeing that same car more and more in your vision. Same thing with a vision board or printed affirmations. They create your reality. I created my vision board about 15 months ago, around the same time as I stated that I was going to go on the Abraham Hicks cruise. Just over a year later EVERYTHING on that board had come to fruition except going to Paris. That is still on the board, and all my boards. I have created a coaching program. I spoke on a few

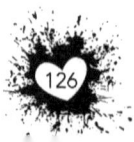

stages. I created Ignite your Power coaching. I created the cruise. I went on vacation. I transformed. You can do the same. Together we can create your vision.

Here are seven key things I think will really propel you into your *Self-Love Journey*

1. **Choose how you start your day**. You can choose to start your day grumpy and irritable or you can choose to start your day grateful that you were given another chance to enjoy life and LIVE.

2. **Get a beautiful journal**, one that you will love to touch and hold every day. Write what you are grateful for in it each night and each morning when you wake up, at least five *different* things. You can also use this journal to write down your feelings, your thoughts, then give them a different spin. It is a great way to see how far you have come when looking back.

3. **Get out in the fresh air every day**, even if it is for a few minutes. Embrace nature all around you. Listen to the birds. Look at the yards. Smell the flowers. Even if you only go around the block, go outside.

4. **Create your vision**. What are your dreams? What are your hopes? DREAM Big. Everything is possible. Everyday visualize for two minutes what you want to create in your life as though it has already happened.

5. **SMILE**. Smiling releases serotonin. When something goes wrong, SMILE. Find the joy, or the positive in in it. You will instantly feel better for being positive and it just may help your bad mood too.

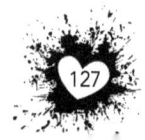

6. **Get Proper Rest**. Lack of sleep can encourage negative thoughts and just may cause you to feel bad. If you are not getting enough rest, a power nap can increase productivity, reset your mood and your focus.

7. **Stay hydrated**. It is so important to keep your muscles and organs hydrated for ultimate performance.

About the Author

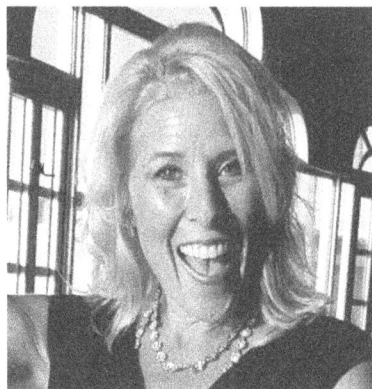

Tiffany Kiefer

Hi, my name is Tiffany Kiefer and I believe in creating happiness and love in all areas of my life. I have been on a self-healing journey for over 20 years, owning several businesses in my quest to find true happiness. With continuously feeling that it was everyone else's responsibility to make me happy, I has finally discovered I could only find it within myself. Through my teachings and coaching practice, I have developed a passion for helping people raise their vibrational level to attract the love, adventure and career they desire and deserve. I am fully committed to inspiring those around me and globally to create the momentum we need in the world to shift the vibration and energy to the GOOD.

You can enjoy my inspiration every weekday morning by going to coffeewithtiffany.net.

You can email me at Riseupnshine777@gmail.com *Follow me on:* Facebook: https://www.facebook.com/tiffany.kiefer Instagram: https://www.instagram.com/tiffany_kiefer Twitter: https://twitter.com/epiphanytifany

Chapter 12

Love Is Who You Are

Linda Evans

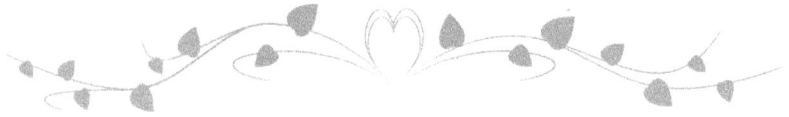

It was about a year after my 15-year-old daughter, Sarah's transition to non-physical when she came to me as spirit as I was walking on the beach. I had been asking Divine Source what it is I must do in order to be "done" in this physical dimension.

I felt like I was on an awakening spiritual path all my life and I had done a good job as a mom in "letting go of my daughter," knowing deeply on a soul level that she is not gone- she is an eternal infinite being with me always. I had been spiritually 'mature' and held the space for her transition as gracefully as possible. I knew of nothing in this dimension that could be more difficult for a parent. I had let go of so many agendas and needs to prove myself or prove anything. I felt really free from most of this dimension's crazy expectations, rabbit holes and insane points of view. I was not suicidal. I just sincerely wanted to know what was left for me to do in this dimension. Sarah spoke to me clearly, as in any conversation you are having over lunch with a friend, telling me that I must learn to love myself fully, freely, fiercely and unconditionally like I had loved her. She added "When you do truly love yourself with every breath and every beat of your heart, you will be experiencing so much joy, you won't be wanting to leave this dimension. You will be having so much fun and feeling the divine love in everything. You will be in awe of the beauty of the planet." She held me with a warm loving energetic hug and continued: "I get to see the beauty of the planet through your eyes. My love for you is flowing always and forever. Your "job" is for you to learn to love yourself with every beat of your beautiful heart." This was not the answer I expected. I had expected a more tangible mission like getting clean drinking water to all people on the planet or being sure all children are loved and fed and have a good clean bed in which to sleep. This new "assignment" surprised and perplexed me. It seemed so simple and clear yet so overwhelming and selfish. How could loving myself be the key that unlocked the experience of true love and joy? I thought it was better to give love than to receive love. How do I receive something from myself? I could not intellectualize this as it made no logical sense. Yet, I felt and experienced so deeply her love in her communication and the "bigger" love to which she was pointing. On a core cellular level, I experienced the heavenly unconditional love essence to which she was referencing. I knew she was pointing toward something beyond my present awareness. I had no idea how I was supposed to experience this deep level of love with every beat of my heart. Yet, I was willing and

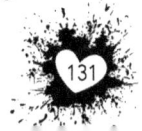

deeply filled with desire and determination to experience that to which she was pointing.

I had no clues as to how this new mission would be accomplished. Was it truly possible? In asking the question, 'How do I love myself unconditionally?,' I began to be shown. First, I was shown all of the judgements which I had about what we had experienced with Sarah. The diagnosis of cancer in my vibrant healthy 13-year-old daughter was bad and wrong. Chemotherapy, radiation and surgery were all bad and wrong. I was a "bad" mother and a terrible spiritual student. I was shown how to let go of these decisions, opinions and judgments which I had created about it all. I began to be willing to see it all differently. I was being shown how to love myself free of all the attachments I had about how anything was "supposed" to happen in life. I was shown how narrow my perspective was and that there is a bigger divine perspective which I couldn't possibly see through the kaleidoscope of judgements I had created. I was desperate to see from that big divine perspective. As I let go of all these personal opinions and judgements from my limited point of view, I was opening up to seeing it all from a different perspective. I was consciously choosing to let go of all of my own opinions and judgements. Every time a judgement came up, I recognized it as a judgment and let it go. Divine spirit was helping me every day. I was being kinder and more gentle with myself. I was being patient with myself. I was getting more massages. I was allowing the grief to flow when it arose. I was spending a lot of time in nature—walking on the beach and feeling the healing love

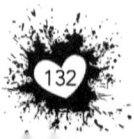

waves flowing at me from the ocean, the wind, the sun, the sand. I was beginning to get a glimpse of a more joyful life.

After months of being kinder and more gentle with myself combined with deep meditation, prayer and self-inquiry, I began to realize that it is less about doing anything and much more about being. I realized that it is not about how, but it is about allowing. As the judgments and pain released from the core of my heart, body, mind and being, I began to experience the flow of the "big" Divine love. I was beginning to remember who I truly am and I was aligning myself with that vibration and allowing more of that to flow through my heart, mind and all the cells of my body, all the nerves and blood vessels. I was letting go of all the rigid thoughts and beliefs which I had about earning and deserving love and about how I thought life should be. I was remembering that love is what I am. Love is my inherent true nature. I was experiencing being in the flow of love and just as one cannot stop the flow of a river, there is no stopping the flow of this Divine love, once you tap into it. As I have allowed more of this love to flow, new neural pathways have been created. It's quite effortless. The harder one tries, the further away it gets. By letting go of the effort of "trying" and just relaxing into a slow deep breath, one can start to get a glimpse of this love which we are. I like to imagine myself sinking deep inside of myself into the ocean of love and well-being that is inside of me. When I rest in that place inside of me, I feel the flow of the love of the universe pulsing through my heart and all the vessels of my body. The more often that I put my attention and awareness on that, the more easily I

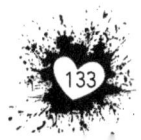

connect to the flow and allow the tap of love to open up and flow more fully and freely. When we are feeling that healing love pulsing through our body, heart, and mind and through all the cells of our body, then it flows outward to others and into all aspects of our lives. Then, when we are sharing this love, we are giving from the overflow and we don't place any conditions or ideas of what we expect to get in return. The flow of love opens up wider and deeper. It just flows out because it can, not with any attachments or hopes about what one will get in return. As we practice this with love and ease, it becomes more natural and grace-filled.

When I walk on the beach, I easily remember that I am love. I see the love flowing abundantly and effortlessly in each wave as it breaks. I feel the love in the wind as it blows open my heart. I smell the love in every flower as it releases the beautiful aromas of the divine and they permeate every cell of my body. I hear the love in every baby's cry as he or she is born into this world and the sound frequencies from the cry vibrate through everything as a healing is experienced by all in the room. I taste the love in every delicious meal I eat as I am so grateful for the beautiful vegetables and resources abundantly gifted to us from Mother Earth. These are just a few of the ways in which I experience the divine love which is truly in everything and everywhere. I invite you to open your heart to the possibility that you are love. I invite you to ask your higher self, or the Divine, or God, or whatever name you like to show you this heavenly love that is inside of you always flowing. I invite you to notice today where you see, hear, feel, smell, taste this essence of love. Allow the universe to show you today this love and it will!

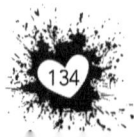

Learning to love ourselves can be difficult if we attempt to do so with the mind. The mind has a lot of conditions that must be met before we can love ourselves. The ego says we must meet certain criteria. For example, we must have the perfect career and the perfect size and shape of body. The mind or ego also insists that you have created the ideal relationship and family—whatever decision the mind has made up as to how the ideal relationship and family looks for you. The mind creates this constant pressure on you with the scenario that you cannot relax and love yourself until all these conditions have been met. It creates the epitome of conditional love and most human beings are under this constant seeking and never really arriving.

Today, I invite you to let go of whatever those drivers are for you which are fueled by the mind and society's expectations. Let go of all the I will happy when.... "I am living in the perfect home," "I have the ideal career," "I have the greatest relationship with the most awesome sex ever," "My body is skinny with the perfect shape." "I have X amount of money in the bank," "I have taken the dream vacation." For some spiritual seekers, it is something like "when I have experienced enlightenment." Take a deep breath and acknowledge the insanity and crazy-making pressure this creates in your life. Give yourself permission to let all those ego "drivers" go and let go of everything you are doing today to try to be good enough to love yourself and let all those associated thoughts, beliefs and emotions go. Consider the possibility of letting yourself just BE. Consider the possibility that right here and now you are good enough and that you are worthy without having to justify anything

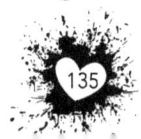

or meet any imposed criteria. Creating goals and intentions can be very helpful in consciously directing energy into your desires. I am suggesting that your goals and intentions be separated from completely loving and accepting yourself. If you are willing to let go of those attachments, then you can sink into the LOVE that you always already are.

If we are always already love, how can it be so difficult to experience this love? Usually, we are the ones who put up the walls, barriers and defenses to love. The fears, insecurities, self-protective walls based on not being good enough can have a stronger vibrational frequency than the love essence vibration, so the fears tend to dominate our vibration. Most of us were not taught how to receive, accept, allow and align with the love that we are. We were taught by parents, teachers and religious leaders that we must be "good" to receive the love. Not only must we be "good" according to their criteria, but if we are not good, we are punished sometimes to the extent that we will likely go the "hell" if we are "bad." As adults, we mentally rationalize that none of this makes sense and we usually reject the concepts we have been taught, yet we often are resisting and reacting to these concepts and spinning in circles. We often feel stuck in this cycle of seeking for love and validation outside ourselves with the peace of self-love and acceptance just outside our reach. After years of trying, we often get frustrated and feel hopeless that we will ever get relief from the crazy rat race of life. Many become exhausted, depressed and just try to make it through each day. Some develop physical symptoms like adrenal fatigue, depression, or other diseases. The

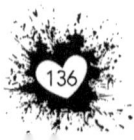

further away from the LOVE that we are we get the more signs and symptoms appear.

Many people also self-medicate with alcohol, drugs, shopping, sex, exercise and sometimes even with spiritual workshops and teachings. These can become addictions when the substance provides temporary relief. The key word here is temporary. The substance can only provide relief for a short while and then even more of the substance is needed. So, whenever you are rewarding yourself after a hard day at work with a drink or whatever your preferred substance is, be sure to ask yourself honestly, is this self-loving or self-medicating? In everything we do, it is insightful to ask this question... Is this self-loving? For example, if I eat this donut or bag of chips, is it self-loving or self-medicating? If I go to the mall and spend $500, is this self-loving? Be honest with yourself, not judgmental. Sometimes the answer will be, yes it is loving, and go for it. Other times, the answer will be, no it is not loving as it will lead to self-sabotage, guilt and self-punishment. It takes some practice to feel into the difference. If we are open hearted and honest, we are often surprised when the truth reveals itself. Our heart always knows the truth in love. I invite you to take a few moments to tune in to "Is this self-loving?" practice on a daily basis.

The more we seek outside, the further away we get from the love that we are. At the core of our being, we are love. Love is our true vibrational essence. Love is our true nature, Love is our home. Love is who we be. These words are pointers-pointing us back inside to ourselves. As we stop seeking for

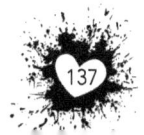

love in "all the wrong places" outside ourselves and make that U-turn back inside ourselves, we encounter the essence of our being. We begin to experience this Love who we be, the Divine, the Inner light, our Inner Being, Higher Self, Divine Grace, Awareness, Consciousness. It does not matter what name you use because the name is also just a pointer. It becomes a bit like the true north on a compass in the woods.

If you feel lost in the dimensions of time and space, place your attention on this deep abiding and unbounded love inside of you and it will guide you home to your center.

Take a deep breath now and relax into this place inside of you where you know you are Love. Rest here for a few minutes and settle into this comfortable place of Love. Say out loud "I am love. I am love. I am love". Notice that you are not just connected to love by an imaginary energy cord in your heart. You are love. Love is vibrating through all the cells of your body. Love is vibrating through your entire heart, your lungs, all the organs of your body, all the blood vessels. Love is pumping through all the arteries and veins in your body. Love is vibrating through your mind and both hemispheres of your brain. You are breathing in love. You are exhaling love.

If thoughts arise saying it can't be so easy, let those thoughts float away like clouds drifting away and dissipating into the sky. Feel this love that you are now through your entire body and being. Make a conscious choice to remember this vibrational frequency essence of love. As you remember this truth of who you are as love, consciously store this memory now in your physical, emotional and mental bodies, know that you can come back into this memory of who you are as love. Know that the more often you come back into this, the stronger will be your vibrational frequency essence of love. It doesn't have to be difficult, in fact it can be quite easy and ease-filled.

You do not have to do anything to be worthy of love. You are always already worthy of love because you are love. When learning and practicing self-love, some people have a difficult time because they feel they are being selfish and they feel it is not loving to focus on self-love.

This can be confusing and create more self-loathing and self-punishment as most sincere people on a spiritual path just want to help others and be of service to others. Learning to accept and allow this love to flow through you completely and without restriction and without "pinching it off" at the source is one of the greatest gifts you can give to others.

By opening yourself up to being a pure vessel of this love and light, you are an invitation to others to do the same. As you are living, moving and breathing in this flow of love, you are sharing this flow of love with those in your life. You can't help but share it. An open valve will flow. Additionally, as you go deeper into the love that you are, you see and feel and know that there is no other. We are all one, so in this awareness of unity consciousness, anything we do to open ourselves up to and accept and receive this true essence of love will benefit everyone with whom we interact. Hence, there is nothing selfish about self-love. Concepts about

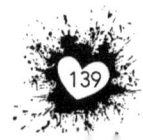

selfishness are just the ego/mind's attempt to manipulate you away from self-love and keep you looking for love outside of you.

All that is required is for us to be in full Allowance of the love that always already is. We are not usually taught this while growing up. We are usually taught to judge and place things in categories of good, bad, right and wrong. All of those decisions literally cut us off from the love. The love is still there, we just can't feel it, see it, or experience it. We become so frustrated and/or depressed because we know at the core of our being that Life is not supposed to be like this. If we are willing to let go of all of our judgments and opinions and barriers to love, and be in Allowance of everything and in judgement of nothing, the love flows infinitely like the waves of the ocean. I have always loved to watch the ocean waves break and I have always been amazed that the waves never ever stop. The waves keep flowing always without effort and with such ease, grace and potency. Amazing waves of love are always flowing to us like this also. For us to experience this Love, we simply let go of our own blocks to this love.

You are likely wondering if it is truly possible to completely love and accept yourself right here and now. YES, it is truly possible. The more you practice, the easier and more comfortable it becomes. There are usually not many examples of others in our lives who are demonstrating this deep vibration of absolute love. Hence, it can feel quite awkward at first. Like anything new, the more you do it the more natural and easy it feels. Just like when we first learn to ride a bike and we needed training wheels to maintain our

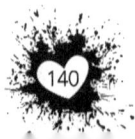

balance, we often need some training wheels when creating new habits and laying down new neural pathways. It is said that 21 days are required to change a habit. If you are in the habit of self judging, self-loathing, putting off self-love until certain criteria has been met and even putting up walls and barriers to love, I invite you to take the next 21 days to let go of those habits and create a new habit of self-love. Look at it like an experiment for yourself. What do you have to lose? Years of beliefs and experiences that block your receiving and allowing of your true nature which is love.

What do you have to gain? Peace which passes all understanding in knowing you are always, already LOVE.

Here's what the 21 Day Experiment in Self-love Looks Like:

You will take 5 to 10 minutes daily to focus on these concepts:

Days 1 to 7: Sit or lie in a comfortable position with your hand on your heart saying quietly and peacefully "I am love, I am love, I am love". Use a timer on your phone to be sure you do this for at least 5 minutes. As the mind comes up with other thoughts, which it will, send them off in cloud to float away and dissipate. After about a minute, you will likely be distracted. Kindly, Gently, Lovingly, bring your attention back to "I am love." Be willing to be this purity of love which you are.

Days 8 to14: Sit on a comfortable chair in front of a mirror with your hand on your heart, say "I Love you. I love you. I

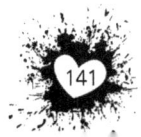

love you." Again, use a timer set for at least 5 minutes as the ego/mind will come up with all sorts of protests and other distractions. If emotions arise, and they will if you are doing this sincerely with your heart wide open, let the emotions flow. This is the dissolving of the past-time walls, barriers, defenses, fences and wounds. Let the emotions release. Love will heal what needs to be healed.

Days 15 to 21: Go outside for a 10-15 min walk and wherever you go and whatever you see say out loud, "I see love. I see love. I see love". If you see mountains, oceans, cars, insects, rocks, say to all you see, "I see love". If something you see seems difficult to acknowledge as love, place your hand on your heart and say it again and again until you feel the shift and you will feel the shift.

Keeping a journal of all that is coming up for you in this 21 Day Experiment can be very beneficial. Be conscious of keeping your heart open. You will become much more aware of when your heart is open and when it is closed by doing this experiment. Placing your hand on your heart invites your heart to open up and allows you to release whatever concept was coming up for you that led your heart to close. This is often a past time heart wound memory of being not good enough, not worthy or even punished. Confusion often arises about the rules and expectations which you were taught as a child. Be gentle with yourself. Be patient and just let it all release knowing that love is the healer and love will heal all wounds if we just let love flow. Be willing to be the love that you always already be.

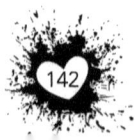

I now know that when my daughter, Sarah, told me that it was time for me to learn to love myself, she was really pointing me toward this remembering that I am this eternal absolute Love always. She was inviting me on this journey of being kinder and more loving to myself which cleared the pathway to see that I am this absolute Love always and forever. I had to surrender all my previous beliefs and concepts about what life is supposed to be and follow my guidance which was taking me back inside of me to this deep profoundly healing essence of love inside of me. The pathway led to this bridge from self-love to there is no "self" to there is only this "big" Love. Life truly is more joyful when you open your heart to experiencing this multi-dimensional Big Love which is always here in us, as us, flowing through us with every breath and beat of our hearts. I invite you to ask to be shown this frequency of love by your higher self. It is always present and available to us. Enjoy the adventures back to you! If you are willing, please let me know how your experiment in self-love is going by emailing me @ loveselfadventures@gmail.com. I would love to hear about your adventures. Imagine a world where everyone remembers and awakens to their true nature as absolute love and awareness.

Will you meet me there?

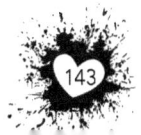

About the Author

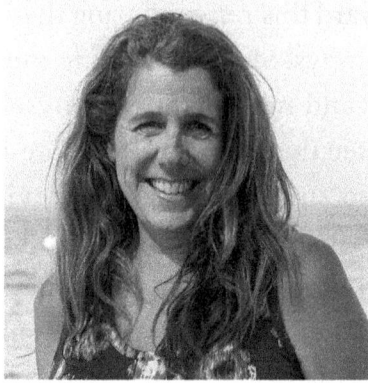

Linda S. Evans

Linda S. Evans, MA, is learning to accept and allow all her life experiences: the good, the bad and the "God-awful" as in the holding space for her precious daughter, Sarah Rose Evans, to re-emerge into nonphysical at the young age of 15 after struggling with a rare form of cancer. Linda has learned to appreciate the depth of learning and expansion of her consciousness which she has experienced as a result of this experience. She continues to harvest the learning and receive the hidden gifts inside this experience.

Linda enjoys providing a safe physical space as well as an energetic welcome to souls as they enter new bodies in her role as a Certified Nurse Midwife. She considers it a deep honor and privilege to have welcomed over 2,000 babies into this 3D dimension.

Linda and her husband, Don, founded a non-profit sanctuary for the celebration of spirit, The Earth & Sky Church in 1999. They provide energy counseling, meditation, and self- healing classes. The intention is to support people in discovering who they are as they uncover and express their own gifts and talents. Linda provides unique facilitation and support for women who desire to let go of limiting beliefs and painful patterns of behavior and ascend into a more joyful way of living and being. Please check out their web site: earthandskychurch.org to see their offerings.

If you desire intuitive, transformational coaching or you would like Linda to provide inspiration at your group event, please contact her at selfloveadventures@gmail.com and be sure to tune in to her podcast, Adventures in SelfLove on i-tunes.

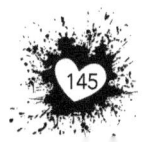

Chapter 13

The Gift of Death

Nikki Jordan

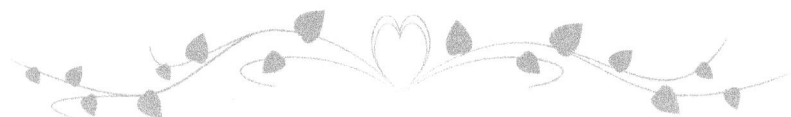

T he puzzle of my life flew apart that day you left, 33 years ago. Afterwards, some things were the same. Some were askew. Some were all together missing. I felt different.

I remember our last conversation only as words. No pictures. I don't know if we were even in the same house. It's funny how we keep memories with the most punch, and the rest turn to dust.

I begged you to join us for my best friend's wedding in Pennsylvania, because at this time in our lives, we saw each other only in summer and at holidays.

No. You were as clear as a 15 ½ year old when choosing between family obligation and beach fun with a friend. Weddings aren't really exciting to boys that age.

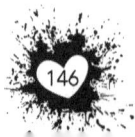

The next time I saw you, you were where they flew you. On that cold metal table at John's Hopkins, an organ donation center for the East Coast. They knew. I knew... at least when I found out where you'd been shot.

All the way in that car ride from our home near D.C. to the hospital in Baltimore, we talked to you. We asked you to make a choice for you - to stay or go. We knew what you loved in life and wanted you to thrive. We also knew how that wouldn't be too possible now that you might suffer living.

Your decision was obvious when I stared into those lifeless marbles. They say eyes are the window to the spirit. And yours had gone right out that hole above your eye.

Your choice to not come to the wedding and your choice to leave unquestionably changed all of our lives. It also granted me a gift for which I'm incredibly grateful. It's one of your greatest marks on me.

Daddy was the one who pointed it out, right after the neighborhood walked out the front door with their empty food bowls from the wake. To this day, I see us standing by the door as those wise words came. *You have the memories of his life, which was a gift. Now, what's the gift in his death?*

That question made me who I am today, likely even fast-forwarded it. I came to know that I didn't fully have all things I thought I did. Like self-love. Thanks to you, I came to know that as a visceral and energetic thing.

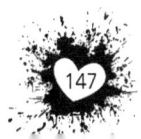

It's likely that anyone in our situation would grasp that we only have this moment to live. The next day, year, or even moment is not guaranteed. So, live life to its fullest and make sure to do what you desire. No regrets. And yet I know people who learned this from loss but did not embody it. To me, not to choose it was to hurt in all the varied dimensions of that word.

For a number of years, living as though I could die came as what others probably saw as flakiness or impatience. I could tack like a sailboat captained by a toddler.

But to me, I chose with what seemed to be an invisible hand pushing me from the back, like the unseen wind that draws a boat forward. Whenever I got an inkling that what I was doing was not my greatest future, or when whatever I'd offered up was done, this hand guided me on.

I came to know this hand as Me - Infinite Me - the one that chose to come here. It pulled on me from a future I couldn't see. *Come here! This will be much more interesting. Come here! We need you. Come here! This you will enjoy.*

Here's a little secret: using this, I've gotten every job I've ever desired so far. That sounds arrogant but I see this a different way. This hand saw what I was looking for that I'd not even known was there. It steered me. And because of this I surrendered to a knowing, beyond the mind that lives in the limited context of this reality.

Each time I followed the pull, I stepped more into Me. As I did so, this cloaked force – this friend – did something

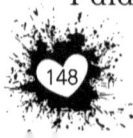

interesting. It pulled *all* of me forward, leaving nothing behind.

I see people leave little bits of themselves everywhere they've been. In yearning and in tethered memories that yank on them. In disappointment and stories. In places and relationships. In anger and worry. And in their convictions.

What if what you were doing next needed all of you in order for you *and it* to thrive? What if the emotional cords you've used to make those memories so vital and significant kept you from fully moving forward? What if you can have memories without all that?

I've come to realize people (myself included) aren't aware they diminish themselves each time they give something significance. You can be aware, care, and act on your convictions, yet the moment you make them solid-real-vital, you use your energy to keep them that way. You diminish your power by depositing some of it in *that* bank.

When people leave themselves places, I sense they often feel weak, scattered, edgy, powerless, anxious, angry, pathetic. Think of how many stories people repeat that drain their greatness. Or the worry they invest in others and issues. Some people never truly create life beyond that, and maybe they don't want to. I just didn't want the pain it caused anymore.

Luckily, I found the reverse is true too and it's just a choice. You can withdraw your power from where you left it and

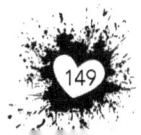

give it back to you. Ultimately loaning your power is neither self-love nor truly empowering to another.

Some people give meaning to loss because they can't imagine a future without what they lost. Or they feel bad, like whatever they lost was meaningless if they do not *show* they care with feeling.

But what if it was just like this: *it was, that happened, it contributed to your life, and now the building blocks of the future are different.* You just can't build a new house with the ashes of the old. It's not strong material.

I knew if I tried to do that it would never make you come back anyhow. I built mine with the gift you gave me.

I learned that self-love is the photo-negative of hurting yourself. We hurt ourselves all the time with our thoughts and feelings, our words and actions – whether we direct them at ourselves or others. We do it without knowing that's what we're doing. Or we get stuck on them, like an addiction.

I know this because I hurt so much when you left. I felt like something was taken out of me.

I discovered I had put some of me in you all those years, calling it love. It was as though I created the definition of me, which included raising you, responsible for you, loving you, having you always there in my life. And when you left, that part of me left too.

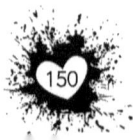

We don't truly understand what we're doing when we love in terms of connection. We put pieces of ourselves in other people's lives, world tragedies, injustices, arguments, problems at work, emergencies. We create cords of significance or control. We become a leaky tire. Never full. Never having *all* of us.

Then one day, I realized that I could call all that energy back, that part of me in you. It was a force that surprisingly came right away when summoned. I felt stronger and whole, clear and free. And I didn't feel I was dishonoring you.

Why? Because somehow, You were still there. Not you in person. You as energy. I know You, and I knew that You were there.

This might sound funny coming from me because you know we never grew up with religion or spirituality. We grew up in the rational world of science. Our world just happened not to have a discussion of God or what was out there, or after here, or even before all this. It wasn't a conversation, just as it wasn't in conversation in many households where parents had let religious affiliation slide and spirituality may have been private.

In this way, I had no dogma. Nothing to release or to hold on to, so as to either validate or invalidate what would become my wildest experiences of Existence.

~~~

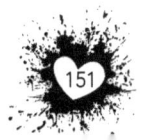

The first casualty of self-love was my first marriage... the one you were supposed to be at, but you died six weeks beforehand. It wasn't that as a newlywed I was lost without you. No, I spent my time with You in your photos in the middle of the night. It was that eventually I saw something in my relationship I had never seen before.

What I thought was a great and deeply loving relationship was in fact finding love IN each other, instead of loving yourself and finding a partner with whom you have fun and ease and adventure. It was the kind of relationship where they say, *They complete each other*. Which apparently meant I missed something in me, so I needed someone else to feel that deep love. Or perhaps we were in love with love. It was a relationship full of feeling.

To be fair, when I leapt toward the next thing, I was truly surprised. It came out of the blue that I would even consider doing life without him.

You know that I never had any substantial work or money until I graduated from college. I'd spent my youth working at home for our family, and I left college with what they said was the highest paying job of any graduate. My new husband and I were paid New York City salaries in a 1980's Atlanta economy. We were more than flush. I felt free.

In Year Two, I wanted a new stereo component, something with full sound. Till then, I'd never had money for fancy. This would be a one-time splurge for fun. For our mutual love of music. He told me he wanted to save money for

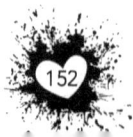

our invisible children in a future that seemed far away, but in which he invented that they would go to private school like he did. I was public school baby. He just didn't see the contribution of this to our living *now*.

We ate turkey legs because they were cheaper. I'd pick at the legs because hate turkey. I don't even eat it at Thanksgiving. And our restaurants were from coupon books. Limited, inexpensive choices.

He won, because we valued love and discussion over fighting. Even though he had inherited several hundred thousand dollars at age 21, he won because planning for a future required practical and logical thought. He won, like he won when "we" decided not to keep the oops-baby a year prior, because it wasn't time. That was the second time I had something taken from me in a year, even if that situation was rationalized.

This is reflection talking. It took me years to see rationality and control for the limitations they are, which is so useful because we all use them in some way – on ourselves and others. But at that time, I don't think I was cognizant of the problem.

All I know is one day I shocked myself and jumped.

~~~

I had applied to graduate school at UC Berkeley. It was a switch of fields from chemistry and business to electrical

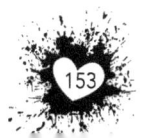

engineering. A stretch, but I saw no problem and for some reason chose only that school.

The day I held the university's envelope in my hand, I was very calm. There were none of the usual butterflies of anticipation. And yet, I knew that if I got in, we'd have to move. He had a good job in Atlanta that he liked, and there was only one other branch of his company in the U.S. In Silicon Valley. It was not Berkeley and we would not be together every day, but it was not far.

As I read the letter, the space around me - the space in which I exist - spread wide. There was no friction, no feeling, only ease.

I knew I was going – my *cells* knew and I could sense it - whether he was going or not. Not choosing for me was not an option. I felt the pull of the Future Me.

The truth never lies. And when you choose from the truth, it feels like total space ... or a comfy sock.

Since then, my greatest choices have involved no plan or agenda; no calculation or pros and cons; no negotiations; no worry of judgment; none of mental-machination-decision-making cognitive stuff.

Cognition is not where self-love lies. Knowing is where.

Why? Because knowing is ease, and ease is the state of self-love. Nothing can sway me when I go there.

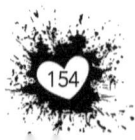

I can't say that my act of self-love didn't affect another. My path diverged before he was even able to follow me across country. I shed long tears for hurting a kind person, but thankfully gratitude has a rear-view mirror.

~ ~ ~

I never told you that several years before you died I had an incredible experience with Existence. I believe this experience maybe even allowed me some ease with your death, because nothing is truly gone. Everything is energy, and all energy is mutable. Most people have to have faith to know that. I had science ... and this.

It was when you were 12 and I was 18. I was sitting in the woods on the steps going down to our community swim club. It was late summer and the DC area crickets were enveloping the world in that 360° surround sound I so love.

My body pulsed for a few seconds with their song, and then all of a sudden - poof! I lost all my skin. My barrier to the world was gone and I was in a black place. Deep in space with all animals, birds, insects, bugs, the forest - everything pulsing as one. One breath, one heartbeat, one motion. One. Not connected. Not interconnected. One and the same.

I was sitting with Garrand, my then boyfriend who later graciously took your place at my wedding after you died. I have no idea how long this experience lasted. Twenty seconds, two minutes, twenty minutes. But what I do know is that time was non-existent. It was All Space.

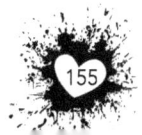

I came back into my skin, once again of this reality and seemingly separate and distinct from what had just been. I asked Garrand if he had felt that. *Felt what?* I explained, and he shook his head with a wide-eyed chuckle. *No, I did not feel that*. I had thought it was a mutual adventure, a gift to us both.

I later came to know that this gift was a thing that monks and seekers spent lifetimes training for, waiting for. That yogis and meditation teachers taught about, but for most of whom I met, it was an external concept; a journey. To me it was something I was IN.

I learned there was a Universe our reality hid.

~~~

Sixteen years later, I called on this Universe to fix my life. Completely frustrated, I walked around Oakland's Lake Merritt and silently screamed, *Show me what I'm meant to do here, or ...*

I didn't finish that sentence because I wasn't going to kill myself, but I just didn't want to be here anymore this way. *Show me or I evaporate*. I was that serious.

It had turned out I was a change agent. In almost every job I had, change was in my wake. Sometimes it was huge, and much of it was not comfortable.

Since I had leapt in Atlanta, I found truth was my compass. On that lake walk, I knew all along I had been working for

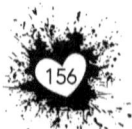

The Organization. Not for the people, not even for those who hired me, no matter how much I liked them. The Organizations had pulled me in for change, and that last one had been most frustrating and painful.

I hurt, and self-love does not hurt.

Two weeks later in Portland, Maine, I missed a movie. Invisible Future Me lured me into the cramped back office of a several-hundred-year-old building. There, a man who later became my teacher plugged me into an intense energy that completely rewired me from head to toe. I couldn't move or speak as the Universe strapped me down so it could unleash my dormant super power. I'd never known anything like it.

Over three years I trained how to use my own power before I worked with others. I went from having four channels to the Universe to eight; then sixteen; then hundreds; then thousands; then hundreds of thousands. And then one day last year - poof! – a total explosion with no number. There is nowhere else to seek anymore, only how to be in this world with the gift of One.

I found my own comfy sock – Infinite Me.

~~~

Since having arrived in Berkeley, I have been in a 31-year relationship. We had both experienced close deaths that shook our hearts, and we both came out fiercely committed

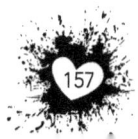

to ourselves (a concept which, by the way, doesn't leave out others).

We never speak much of our reasons for being together. Nor do we often say, *I love you*. Our relationship is based on being You as the most vital thing. It is what attracted us in the first place.

We hate drama; the fight hurts. When we are hurting ourselves or each other, we point it out. We have each other's back more than we have our own. The moment one of us goes off true north, the other steers them back to full power.

We are trained in the rational world yet we both operate off of knowing, even if we temporarily doubt ourselves. We have faith that the Universe watches over us, and our lives are storybooks of this many times over.

We are not the same ... and yet we are. And when we have tough times, I usually don't fear. Why? Because You taught me to choose Me and everything will work out.

In this relationship, we just know the moment we stop enjoying each other and doing the adventure of life together, things could change. We live with the ease and space of that truth because birth, change, and death are the only things guaranteed.

At yet I always remember that *I knew* ... the moment I met him. It felt like I put on a comfy sock, a space of nurturing and ease, just like when I had you in my life all those years.

Choosing this was self-love.

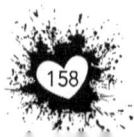

About the Author

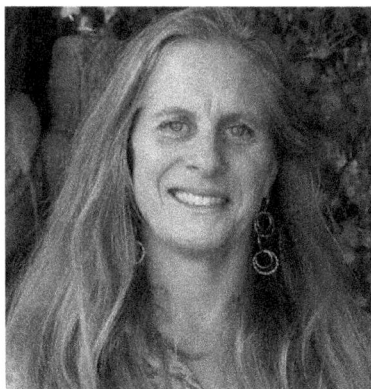

Nikki Jordan

Nikki Jordan is a gifted energy healer who had no idea she was one. Her life's work has been to create the change that's being asked for. Until she knew that, she thought she was just on a random and fun adventure.

She is a consciousness facilitator and a body whisperer. Over twenty years she has practiced and taught consciousness, energy work, Yamuna® body rolling-foot fitness-face ball, TRE® stress/trauma release, Access Consciousness®, reflexology and yoga. Her former career was in science, engineering and business. You can learn more about Nikki at her website www.healthyandrested.com.

Chapter 14

A Journey to Me

Minette "The Energist"

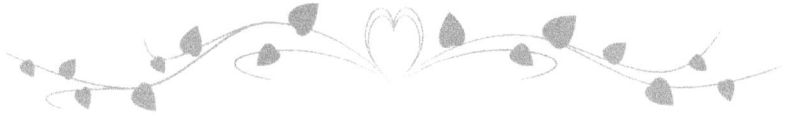

Love is a vibration, it's our Natural Essence, it's when our heart, mind and soul are in alignment. It's divine beauty that lies in being ourselves and starts with self-love.

I love and accept who I am unconditionally. I give and receive love freely, fully and deeply. However this has not always been so and took me years to say. I suffered great trauma and adversity in my life, was treated unkindly and cruelly by those that I loved most, often made to feel less than or unworthy, never good enough. I accepted this as my truth for quite some time (even though deep inside I knew something was not quite in alignment). I knew there had to be more to life. I know now, that I am what they call an empath. Today this is a gift, in my early life it was a curse, I could feel other people's pain and emotions as if they were my very own. I could not understand how people could be so cruel and unkind to each other especially those they claim to love. I spent much of my early years trying to

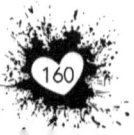

ease people suffering at my own expense, always giving and giving, running on fumes but unable to say no to someone in need. I found this to be an unhealthy pattern, people would feel better after being around me, they could tell me their life stories so easily with no judgment, I found them leaning on me for their happiness. And while everyone was leaning on me, I had never felt more alone, *I created a space* where I had no one to lean on, no one to care if I was happy. This left me chronically ill and in a constant state of anxiety, frustration, anger and at times longing for an end to it all. I knew something had to change. Hence began the path of self-discovery, self-acceptance and self-love. Believe me when I say, if I can do this and choose this journey of self-love to discover the possibilities of ME, anyone can. I share with you now the awareness's, wisdom and tools that allowed me to choose "Me".

When I first began this journey, I had no idea how beautiful the gift of Me could truly be. I like so many others had been programmed since birth with limiting beliefs and thought patterns, that self-love is selfish, I was taught to sacrifice and serve the needs of others first and my own needs last, if ever. I realized I had taught people how to treat me through my actions and choices. I taught them I am only here to serve, I will sacrifice my happiness for yours and I come last. This space I created was a great unkindness to everyone. For we are not here only to serve, we are here to contribute and how much more can we contribute when our cup is full. But so many of us, myself included chose for years to run around with my cup empty, my body and soul on fumes and put others first. I had hit the bottom and was ready

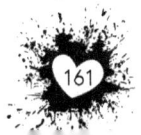

for change. I started with setting boundaries for myself, by learning to say no to those that were what I call energy drainers. I know it sounds simple, but it was one of the most difficult things that I'd ever done. It was hard to tell someone no, but I knew it was required. I had created a reality, or comfort zone (A place I now refer to as the discomfort Zone, because if it was that comfortable we would not be longing for change), that was comfortable for everyone else but me, as they relied on me for their happiness, (And we all know where that leads everyone blames you, and is rarely happy, because happiness is an inside job that one can only choose for themselves).

Many around me were not happy that I was saying no, some even told me I was being selfish. However difficult it was in the beginning it became easier and lighter the more I chose to create these healthy boundaries. And miraculously the side effect of this choice was that those who had depended on me started to build different support systems and felt empowered to create their own happiness. I realized then that allowing them to depend on me, was keeping them from choosing to create their own happiness. I had the awareness that if we are always the one fixing things for others and making them feel better, they sometimes struggle to know that they can find solutions to their own challenges. My choice to put me first was inspiring them to choose to put themselves first. This choice to create these boundaries allowed me for the first time, to have some time for myself.

Now with time to reflect and look inside of myself, I started to identify thoughts, feelings and emotions that carried a

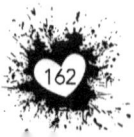

heavy charge or energy. I learned that a memory without an emotional charge is wisdom. I begin clearing the charges of my past and chose to forgive. I realized living in the past and carrying these dense thoughts, feelings and emotions around, were only hurting me, and I was ready to stop hurting. When we forgive it is for ourselves not others, as we release these energies we open our heart to allow more love and light in.

"You only have to forgive once. To resent, you have to do it all day, every day." ~ ML Stedman

While I was releasing and forgiving, I started to also forgive myself. I often, like many others got caught up in self-judgment and negative self-talk (which often stems from other people's insecurities and opinions)," I'm not good enough", "I'll never have that", "why would anyone want me". I found myself in this pattern so many times, but it just took committing to me (and I hope for you committing to yourself) to start to undo this programming and thought process. I had made other people's opinions more important than my own. I'd let their opinions cause harmful thoughts. I shouldn't even say cause harmful thoughts because we have free will and choice as to what we give significance to. I stopped making other people's opinions more valuable than my own. This created a significant change in my inner dialogue. For now when I find myself having a negative thought, I am able to redirect it. I ask myself when experiencing a thought or feeling that is not comfortable, is this contributing to the life I truly desire and to me continuing to love myself? If the answer is no, I redirect

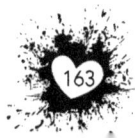

and shift my thoughts and energy to that of gratitude for all that I do have. This allowed me to gain some control over my thought patterns. Because our mind is a muscle and the more we use it and choose us, the easier it gets until those thought patterns, are gone and new ones that contribute to us are created. This gratitude for everything that I've chose to cultivate, has allowed me to release victim thinking and limitations and choose me. More of me then I'd ever known before, as a creator and a thriver not only a survivor. From this new space and reality I have chosen to create I now have a life filled with love, friendship, and so many blessings. I share with you now a few of my favorite things that remind and inspire me to continue to choose love and some more clarity on the tools that facilitated my new reality.

Quotes

"To be beautiful means to be yourself. You don't need to be accepted by others. You need to accept yourself" ~ Rumi

"Your task is not to seek for love, but merely to seek and find all the barriers within yourself that you have built against it"
~ Rumi

"To love oneself is the beginning of a lifelong Romance"
~ Oscar Wilde

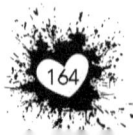

Breathwork

Close your eyes and take a deep breath, focusing on your heart. Visualize breathing love in (through your nose) and exhaling (from your mouth) lower energies and densities that are weighing you down.

Self-Love Affirmation

Say out loud (or to yourself if you prefer) I love and Accept myself fully and freely just as I am. I Love and Accept who I Am unconditionally. I receive and show love freely, fully and deeply. I am valuable and worthy of love. Love flows to me freely and in abundance. My heart is filled with love and shines on those around me. I am embraced by the loving energy of the universe. I am LOVE. Repeat until you start to feel lighter.

An inspirational poem can change your energy. I choose: As I Began to love myself by Charlie Chaplin. "As I began to love myself I found that anguish and emotional suffering are only warning signs that I was living against my own truth. Today, I know, this is AUTHENTICITY. (for complete poem go to goodreads.com/quotes)

More Tools for Choosing Self-Love

Create healthy boundaries and identify energy drainers. You know those people that come around and leave you feeling empty. Time to put an end to these toxic relationships regardless of who they are. I now choose relationships

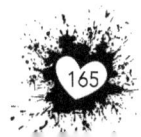

not *bound by blood, but created with love*. This meant for me whether someone was related to me or not, I no longer allowed them to treat me unkindly. If you have people in your life that always make you feel less than, it's time to stop listening to them and become your own advocate and savior. Because the most important opinion is yours. Know you are worthy of love, demand for yourself love on all levels. I found it to be true with my own experience and that of many of my clients that we can only receive the level of love we are willing to give to ourselves. Take that in for just a moment, it means that even if the *perfect* person came along and loved us unconditionally we could not receive this and would either have to sabotage or make it wrong in some way. Self-love is kind, nurturing, gentle, it is truly and unconditionally loving and accepting , *Who You Are Now* (not an idea of who you think you need to be). It's about gaining an appreciation for your creation of YOU. It is vital to our inner peace and happiness. Once we truly accept ourselves we can come to a place where we can grow and embrace our true essence and the true gift we can be to ourselves. And it's not so much about learning this, it's about remembering. Be the first one in line to love you unconditionally, because if you cannot love yourself unconditionally how can someone else. Make love internal first. Be love and it will flow to you.

Redirect your thoughts. When you're experiencing thoughts that are not a contribution to your happiness, change lanes. I know this sounds funny but if we looked at our thought patterns as routes we can choose a smooth happy ride or a bumpy traumatic ride this is our choice, we create our reality. Shift your thought s to gratitude for that which you

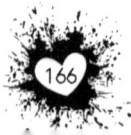

do have, science has shown that an attitude of gratitude can literally shift the molecular structure of your brain and heart. When we start to master this, life becomes so much easier, as if we go from swimming upstream fighting the current to gliding to our desired destination with the universe on our side. So become your own cheerleader, because if you cannot be on your team why would anyone else want to.

Forgive others and yourself. Release the anger from within, this allows more room for love. Forgive yourself because there is no failure only feedback. You have never done anything wrong, only made decisions based off of your current level of awareness and consciousness at the time. Now from the space of forgiveness and acceptance, you have the wisdom and feedback to create better choices and possibilities for your future.

Start identifying and setting goals that can bring more of what you desire into your life. Find the things that fill your heart with light and work towards those. It's key in this step to have your goals be towards rather than away from. *Instead of focusing on what you survived focus on what you can create/ conquer now.* For example, when I first started setting goals I proclaimed, no one would ever abuse me or treat me the way my family did. The energy of this is an away from. I was focused on my past as a thing to get away from and not to repeat, instead of creating my future as I would like it to be. Now with a new level of awareness and conscious choice my goal is now phrased, I desire a life filled with love, joy, prosperity and gratitude for everything. Now the energy of this is towards creating my future and not escaping my past.

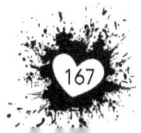

This is vital so we can begin to see and envision our desired future and not anchor to the past with victim energy.

Empowering actions daily, just for you just for fun you don't have to share it with anyone unless you choose. Examples of empowering actions are painting, dancing, meditating, affirmations, taking a walk in nature, buying yourself flowers, journaling and reading. Explore your spirituality, find and choose things that lighten your spirit and fill your heart with joy. Let your creativity and passion flow. Your reality shows where your energy flows.

These tools and my choice to commit to loving myself unconditionally have allowed me to flourish and expand. I now contribute from a wondrous space of love, gratitude and kindness. With my heart full, I know anything is Possible!! Choosing to share this with those in the world that are READY FOR CHANGE, I've built a successful and rewarding practice facilitating others around the globe on their journey of discovering and choosing self-love, so that they can create the life they are meant to live.

When you're around someone who truly loves them self not from the ego but from the heart, its magnetic and it's an invitation to us all, to know it's possible, and to choose to be our beautiful genuine selves, this is our true essence, our fundamental truth is LOVE. So be the change and LOVE you want to see in the world!

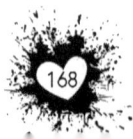

About the Author

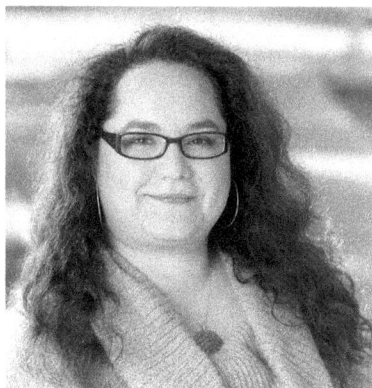

Minette "The Energist"

International best selling author, consciousness facilitator and Transformational Empowerment coach Minette "The Energist" has dedicated her life to assisting people shift their mindsets and clear the energies that are holding them back from creating the life they truly desire. A life filled with more joy, love, prosperity and receiving of ALL the gifts we all possess inside. She was led to this path while searching for tools to help her overcome her own traumatic abuse filled childhood and an accident that almost left her paralyzed. While being labeled a "Survivor" by society, she knew that there was something else possible, so began the road to Enlightenment and a path from "Survival " to "Thrival". This path lead to becoming a Reiki Master, Theta Healer, Quantum Healer, Seraphim Angel Healer, Intuitive Card Reader, Master Abuse Healer, Reconnective Healer, Ayurvedic Mudding Therapist, Aromatherapist, Access Consciousness Bars/ Body Process/Facelift Facilitator, EFT (Emotional Freedom Technique) Practitioner, Hypnotherapist, Certified Professional

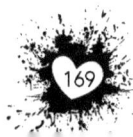

Life Coach, NLP (Neurolinguistic Programming) Certified Coach, Timeline Therapist and several other modalities. All these and having an opportunity to study with doctors from around the world, has led to Minette having a large toolbox that allows her to facilitate people to transform their life. So if you are truly ready for change, and to choose YOU, schedule your creation of possibilities session today!!

www.Minette.world

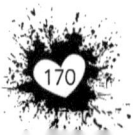

Chapter 15

The Power of Loving Yourself

Kaarin Alisa

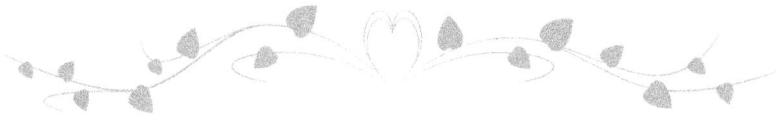

You are divine. You have a divine purpose for being here. If you've lost your connection to that divine spark, the world seems more like a battlefield, than a home. But the world doesn't have to be a battlefield. It can be a giant playground with everything you need to play, in the way you want to play, right at your divine fingertips.

I know, because like you, I've lived it. I couldn't give myself the love, honor, and respect I deserved. I allowed the fallout of daily battles keep me from experiencing the love of life and self that is my divine birthright.

But at some point, I said "NO MORE!" The pleas for help emanating from my core caught my attention. The choice

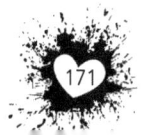

was simple, either I create a new life, or I end this life and hope for better in the next incarnation.

If you've ever fallen into this pit of despair, you know the choice I refer to. And even if you haven't fallen so far, you're reading this book because you realize you're in an old paradigm that you want to change. You're here because you want to find the playground again – to allow your spirit to guide you to the best life you can create.

Loving yourself is the vehicle to that life.

The power unleashed when you fall in love with the divine, indestructible you at your core, is the key to shifting your life away from the battlefield and onto the playground. It's a not-so-subtle shift of perspective; an acknowledgement of your divinity. It's a step worth taking.

Take off your battle fatigues, for just a little while, and explore what I've learned that can help you make this not-so-subtle shift of consciousness from embattled to deeply loved.

Make a Commitment

First things first; make a commitment. Even if you don't believe it now, tell yourself that whatever you've been blind to, you'll illuminate; that you're ready to live with the respect, honor, and love that you truly deserve.

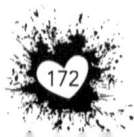

Tell yourself here and now that you're grateful to your body, mind, and spirit for hanging in with you all these years; that you're grateful to have them with you now. Ask them to be your allies on this journey.

And lastly, know that what you commit to you can achieve. It doesn't matter what any of the yesterdays were like, you're free in this moment to take a new path, make a new pact with life, and love yourself for who you are, here and now.

Commit. Accept the end goal.

When you truly love yourself, you'll display the characteristics of empathy, love, and generosity of spirit. You'll be attractive to things you deem worth attracting. Life will bring you joy and surround you with like-minded people. And when you truly love yourself, you'll wonder at how you survived without this powerful friendship forged with your own divine spark.

Insight #1

What you judge in others is what you cannot accept about yourself

We live in an illusion designed to give us an experience we call life. The world is a big mirror. What you judge or hate about yourself, what you cannot accept about yourself, you'll see in other people and you'll judge them for it. It's also true that what you're *afraid* you are, or *afraid* you're becoming, you'll see in other people and judge them for it.

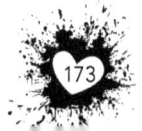

173

The world will help you see yourself even if you turn a blind eye to yourself, because truth is persistent.

Gautama Buddha put it like this: "Three things cannot be long hidden: the sun, the moon, and the truth."

When you refuse see the truth of who you are, you force your truth to make itself known through the external world. For the sake of truth, the world is placed in the position to mirror you back to you. So when you're looking at that mirror, you see in it, the parts of you and your fears that you've been blind to.

Exercise: Pick a person you've judged harshly. Write down the characteristics you judge in them. Assess what bothers you about their behavior, or looks, or life choices. Now rewrite each item in the first person as it might apply to you. Example: If you wrote you judge your sister for being bossy, look at your own life. Are there people you're being bossy to? Include how you act toward yourself. You may see that you go out of your way not to be bossy like her. The rewrite might be, "I'm afraid of being bossy." Do this with at least five people you've judged and see if you find common threads.

Tip: With each exercise, perform it several times over days, until you feel you've uncovered something you previously didn't see about yourself. And it's alright to revisit exercises as your paradigm shifts.

Insight #2

What you resist you become

I could also say it this way: What you resist you think about, and what you think about you become. What you put your attention on will be reinforced and multiply.

- What are you holding onto so tightly that it must stay with you?
- What do you hate about yourself that no matter what you seem to do, it's all you see, all you know, all you think about?

When I was a teenager, I learned how to ride a bicycle in an elementary school playground. Each time I began to ride, I smacked into one of two tetherball poles. The playground was obstruction free, aside from these two poles, but I couldn't avoid hitting them. Why? Because I was so afraid of hitting them, the idea of not hitting them was the only thing I could think of. In my fear, my every thought was to NOT hit the pole, so of course I hit the pole.

It's an exact metaphor for what you resist, you become. I resisted the pole so forcefully, I had no choice but to bring it to me.

- What are you resisting in your life?
- What are you drawing to you?
- What are you becoming simply by virtue of the fact that you are at war with the idea of it?

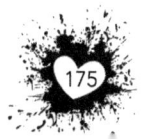

Exercise: You have five minutes to describe yourself. Use whatever language pops out first. Don't second guess yourself. You want to capture your working impression of yourself as it comes out of you unadulterated. Don't think about what your thoughts mean.

Now, look back over this list and separate them into desirable and undesirable traits. Do any of the traits you deemed undesirable mirror traits you identified in the exercise for insight #1? Are there any other patterns or ah-ha's you can see in this list?

Tip: When you find things about yourself or others that you judged erroneously, remember to do a forgiveness exercise to begin the healing process.

Insight #3

What you resist will persist

Another way to say this is what you fight for you get to keep. Resistance of a thing is a form of fighting that thing.

You can probably relate to this idea by thinking of something you desperately wanted to change about yourself only to find that at the end of your journey, instead of releasing what you didn't want, it was more firmly entrenched. Perhaps you wanted to lose 10 pounds and when you were done waging war on your body, you gained back 15.

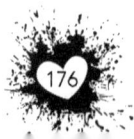

Habits and other behaviors and states can be changed, but not through fighting them, but rather to replace them with something new. Instead of fighting, release and replace.

Another way we resist something is to fight for it with our words. The person who says, I can't instead of I can. For example, perhaps you want to increase memory, but instead of affirming that your memory expands, you say things that affirm the opposite, like: 'My memory is so bad,' or 'I'll forget what you just said,' or, 'count on me to forget where my car is parked.'

- What are you resisting?
- What internal war are you waging that keeps you from achieving – keeps you from experiencing your dreams?

Listen to your words for big clues. Do you ever hear yourself say, 'This always happens,' or 'Every time I...' How about, 'I try, but it just doesn't change.' These black and white statements indicate you are resisting and fighting.

You can work mighty hard to convince others that you are who you are because of what happened to you, or how you were born, or what someone did to you long ago. But it's rarely the truth in your present.

Exercise: Be courageous. Think about, who have you convinced of your plight? What are you fighting against so hard you get to keep it? What are you fighting for that, if you stopped fighting for it, it might go away? Who or what

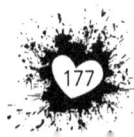

in your support system are you in danger of losing if you change your story?

Tip: Be honest and open with yourself, or an alliance with your inner-self will be difficult to forge. Take responsibility for who you've been, so a new you can emerge.

Insight #4

You only accept what you 've been exposed to AND are in agreement with

Another way to say it is that your mind frames your life by selecting your experiences based on the criteria you give it.

Your brain engages in a process of severe selectivity. Information streams into your being at an overwhelming rate. There are perhaps 20,000 things happening in any minute, from colors, movement, temperatures, people, how many times you breath, how fast your heart is beating, sounds, ideas, thoughts; it's flying in at a rate you cannot handle unless you are selective.

The brain selects what to pay attention to based on criteria you give it. You have the option and power to give your brain new criteria. It's critical to give your brain criteria about what kind of people you want to be around, and what kinds of experiences you'd rather have.

Up until now, without even thinking about it consciously, you gave your brain judgmental and painful criteria. You gave this criteria to your brain every day, over and over.

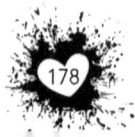

So, when the billions of daily signals came rushing in, your brain looked over the criteria list and said something like, 'Ok, I'll notice anything that tells me I'm... unworthy of love. Check!' Fill in the details with your own judgments of self.

The point is you make up the criteria based on the story you tell yourself. Your brain doesn't know any better. It's an obedient helper. It sees what you think about and therefore frames your perceptions based on what it assumes is important to you.

And when your perceptions change, your experience of the world automatically changes in response

Exercise: Pay attention to what you notice for 24 hours. Make note of any patterns you see. Then, for the next 24 hours, see if you can shift your perspective to notice things you might have dismissed before. In this exercise, make you and your desired experiences a priority.

Tip: You have permission to be selfish in what you look for.

Insight #5

Self-love is recognition of your own divinity

When you accept yourself for who you truly are, you recognize the divinity of your true self.

Earlier in my life, waking up each day felt like coming out of a dream into a nightmare. I thought the divine had forsaken me. But the joke was on me, because I was right. I had fallen

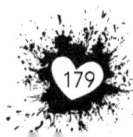

out of favor with the divine that lives in me; this brought me doubt, confusion, hatred, judgment; all the things I didn't want.

But when I gave that up, and saw myself standing as a divine being, I was free to embrace the real me. Can you, because like me, you're part of the divine and doesn't divinity deserve all the good things? All the pleasure? All the joy? All the love?

You carry a spark of all-that-is within you. Surrender to it. From this place of surrender, you can begin to feel true love for yourself, the world, and everything in it.

Exercise: Go to https://bit.ly/2RyaOnW and download a PDF set of affirmation cards designed to help you see yourself, and therefore the world, in a new way. They can help you uncover the self-love you were born to embody.

Tip: print and cut these sheets into cards so you can place them around you or pull them out of your pocket when you need a lift or change of perspective.

Let's Play

You are divine. You have a divine purpose for being here. Today you will sow new seeds of consciousness and walk into your future committed to loving yourself. The world you live in isn't a battlefield, it's a giant playground, and everything you need to play, in the way you decide to play, is right at your divine fingertips when you let yourself be loved from within. Embrace the true you – it's time to play!

About the Author

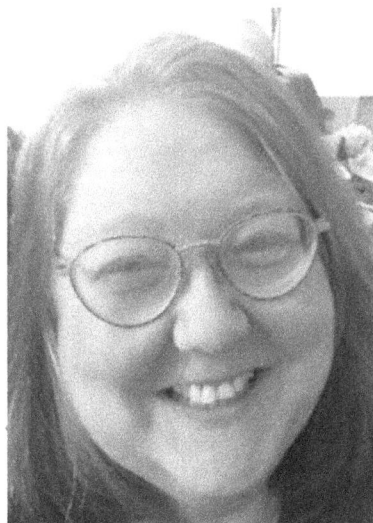

Kaarin Alisa

Author, Teacher, and Metaphysician

Kaarin is a catalyst for spiritual growth and personal transformation. She has honed her abilities as a change agent in the metaphysical and energetic arts for more than forty years, practicing as a spiritual adviser, clinical hypnotherapist, teacher, and energy practitioner.

Kaarin is passionate about higher consciousness and her inner calling is to help humanity raise the collective consciousness by helping as many people as possible raise their individual consciousness. To this end, Kaarin has forged a lifelong relationship with Yeshua (Jesus) and has honed the ability to interact and collaborate with him through both her own personal development and her work with others seeking guidance. Her bestselling book written with Yeshua called "Journey of a Prophet: Jesus Tells His Story," is in its second edition.

International bestselling author and sought-after speaker, Kaarin offers tele-seminars, workshops, and private sessions by appointment.

http://kaarinalisa.com
http://yeshuasays.com
http://journeyofaprophet.com

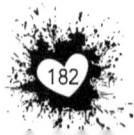

Chapter 16

As a Lotus Flower Blossoms

Erica Glessing

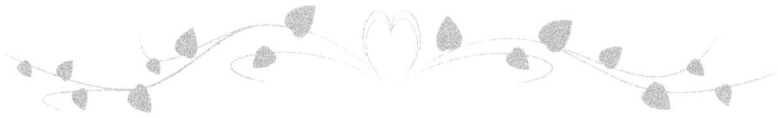

In this connectivity with all that is joy, the world opens up as a lotus blooms.
I am the lotus bud.

I am the lotus partially open, shyly breathing some of heaven's light.

I am the fully expressed and blossomed lotus.

And, I am the once-was-a-lotus now ready for the next journey.

Life is creative expression for me. As I allow more new expressions of me to evolve, I am so curious what I will be doing or saying next. It is the infinity of me that I treasure.

It is belonging in a dark night club after hours, the only white person for miles, dancing with the rhythm of me -- this is one aspect of me. The RNB hip hop music lover of me.

The mornings, when I rise, I write. It is these waking moments of poetry where I write and dance to gospel, this is me too.

In the later mornings, the business mogul of me, where I build empires. This is the web-savvy business owner of me, where I can see in my mind's eye what will unfold and focus my energy right where the sweet juice will be flowing.

It is the mom of me, the mom who will leave all the other callings to tend to my flock of three beings I invited to be here with me as my children this lifetime. The mom of me is imperfect as can be, and delights in each of the kids as they go through the dips and heights of childhood.

I know I confuse people because they are looking to see "Who are you?" and perhaps it would be less confusing if I were the tiny lotus bud not yet formed. Or the brightly bloomed lotus fully sharing all of my gifts and potency. In truth I am all of this, and more.

Even the children of me, my trio of beautiful beings, even the children of me are a fragment of the whole of me. Some days it seems they are my all, other days I see them turn into their own lotus blossoms -- and make their own way into the world, in its glorious perfection.

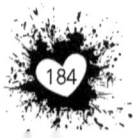

It would be more comfortable indeed if I were one simple flower the same and yet, that would be a silk flower. I can't be a silk flower. I could try and try to go back to become a silk flower, to be the same each day, and this would never actually be my essence of me.

Each day I wake, I stare into the eyes of mine that are a green blue purple and change colors, for I have eyes that change colors, and I get this essence of the greater spirit of me. Not every person has eyes that change colors!

As a young child, I was given a clue of me when I began to ride horses at age three. I love to ride fast, ski fast, dance fast, love fast. At age three I could read captions in Time Magazine (according to the parents of me). Then at age six I could read full books and was always placed in front of the class to read to my fellow first graders in elementary school (Berkeley California).

At age 12, we were living in Palo Alto, California and I discovered the dance of me! Oh! I discovered the music and dance of me! I danced with a teacher who gave us great freedom to move and express ourselves in ways I had not chosen previously. Now at age 14, my first poems were published in a book of other poets at Palo Alto High School. The poem of me was born, and this light would brighten other's lives for decades and decades.

The courageous journey for me was going back to the me of me. The changing eye colors of me. The languages I learned like breathing — Japanese, Chinese, French,

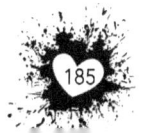

Spanish -- I stopped there, I would have been content to learn languages every year forever. I stood up and chose to be bigger rather than smaller – to love deeper rather than less – to reach for the stars and connect with Heaven for my faith is stronger than the roaring ocean.

I believe when you take time to look into your own eyes, you will see such mystery that you may become uncomfortable. You might want to try to become something, generate a fabulous career, like an attorney, or a dentist, or maybe an engineer. A name on you will give you comfort, and yet, it can also give you chains. It is wonderful to be this, this name of a career of you, and yet, do not confuse a career with your entire being!

You are magic.

Behind the writer, poet, magic language learner, dancer, animal whisperer, I asked myself again.

"Who Am I?"

This seeking to name oneself can be quite wild. I had fun this year and created a new social media identity. The funny thing was it didn't mask me that much. Within a few weeks, I was already being seen differently than the rest. A bright light cannot truly be dimmed.

People can get very frustrated with trying to get who I am. I remember one friend said as we were roller skating to music

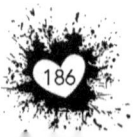

"You are hard to follow, I never know what moves you will take next."

People do seek to follow, because the validation of being a unicorn is possibly daunting. Each of you is a unicorn, each of you is magic. Each of you cannot fully be defined.

How do I validate the moon, the sun, the stars, the night sky? How do I validate the magic of asking to manifest and having it all manifest?

Getting Lost

On this journey I get lost. It's so sad! I get lost behind living in the wrong place and marrying the wrong person and burying myself in debt so big it would be easier to die than fund everything to clear my name.

It is so bitter and so sweet, this lifetime. I most certainly do not have the answers. I am however, willing to ask questions.

Not Alone

I'm going to go back to the beginning now and look at the journey of a lotus flower. From a seed to a closed bud to an open flower, mystical in its journey, beautiful for no reason other than its beingness. Let's say a sun ray was too hot one day and burned a dark circle on one petal of the flower.

Is the flower now less beautiful, for the marring scar? I contend the flower is no less beautiful. It has just been

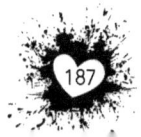

through a day of scorching heat when the sun's rays got through the protective coverings and left its mark.

And so are the exes, the ones who didn't stay, the ones who left marks but could not hold back the ultimate beauty of my essence. For spirit is effervescent. Spirit keeps raising its face to the sky.

Each has a dance, and none is alone. It is all of us dancing together that gives our world form and function.

It is the creative expression of beingness that you truly are, at your essence.

Sometimes I am asked "How do I know if my creation is original enough?"

I laugh. I know, that is not very reverent. I laugh! I say, "How do you know if your fingerprint is unique enough?"

Your voice, your story, you are indeed one individual snowflake, one individual footprint on sand. You came here to express and to appreciate yourself, and this is the courageous self-love journey.

It is not for the meek, perhaps. For as I stare into my own green or blue or purple eyes, I know that there will not be another me like me, another child born in the 1960s, raised in Berkeley, then Palo Alto, raised in a culture of change and education.

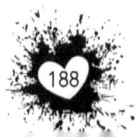

For this very me of me, this uncovering of the petals to seek my core, this is the journey that I chose when the seeds of my parents came together, and I looked down from spirit and said "Oh! I'll take that body!"

And I chose a very curvy Italian Irish German body with light eyes and dark coloring, and my hair could be any one of a number of different ethnic descents -- I love to be near people whose skin is different from mine, whose eyes are different from mine -- and I also love to be near people who are different ages from my age.

It is this curiosity that keeps my journey fresh.

The Role of Forgiveness

To you I would say, forgive yourself for your courageous self-love journey. Forgive yourself for your fumbles. Forgive yourself for your brilliance. Forgive yourself for outshining other flowers who bloomed before you or who may die never having bloomed, at all.

When you are stuck, go and look at yourself in the mirror. Tune into your eyes. See what you see when you look in your eyes. It's a magical place, and you do reside where the universe lies.

All of the universe is within you, and you are a dancing frequency of light given to mankind to change the world.

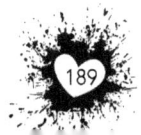

It may not be easy, every day. It's worth it, though. Express the love of you, the wisdom of you, the laughter of you. Overcome your weaknesses and to learn to trust your strengths — this is all a valuable journey.

I love one poem by Maya Angelou particularly "And Still I Rise." It's about rising up, even in the face of adversity.

Recently my dear friend DeAnna read spirit to me from messages of the late Dr. Martin Luther King, Jr. He shared that we (collectively) would begin collectively as a culture to lose so much focus on form and connect bigger to spirit in the years to come. He shared that light will reign, and we are all perfect, now here on earth and in the future, and on the other side.

May you learn to trust that all is well.

All is well.

Truly.

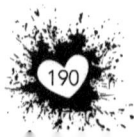

About the Author

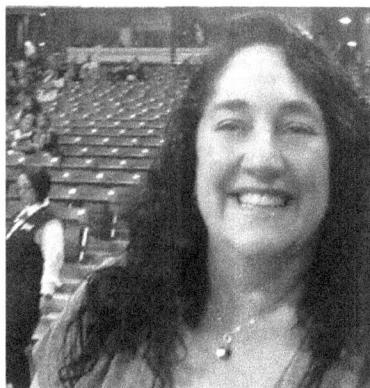

Erica Glessing

Erica Glessing writes books and poems. Erica believes when you tell your story, you change the world. She has penned or edited 34+ #1 bestselling books. Erica has a podcast called "The Erica Glessing Show."

She runs the Happy Communications Group, inclusive of Happy Publishing, Happy2LeadGen (hyperglobal omnipresence) Palo Alto SEO and Lead Generation (hyperlocal omnipresence), Podcast Passion, a podcast production done-with-you program, and is ghostwriting some insanely powerful books.

Erica believes in you. All the stages of you, and wherever you are on this life journey.

You can tune into her podcast at www.TheEricaGlessingShow. com.

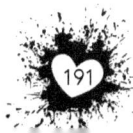

Bonus

Joshua T. Osborne

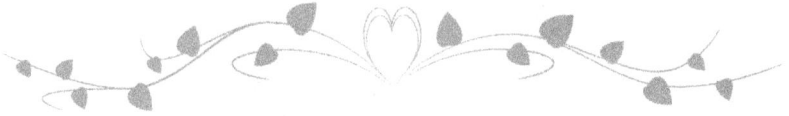

A n Excerpt from a new book soon-to-be-released by
Joshua T. Osborne on his journey from being locked
up in a cell to living a life of Colorado Luxury.

Excerpt...

I was nine when I committed my first crime.

It got worse.

At 21, I was in solitary confinement where I lived 23 hours
locked up in a cell by myself, 30 minutes in the gym, and
30 minutes to shower.

Jail could have made me a better criminal, or a better man.
I chose the latter. Here's a look into the changes and how
I came to be married, with two beautiful sons, living in a
neighborhood in Colorado I could never have imagined,
with faith, family, finance and fitness thriving.

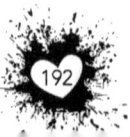

I don't blame anyone but me for my life. And now as I drive up into my own home in my choice of cars, I do not take one moment for granted.

I can blink and be back, locked up, 13 felonies, busted, and running with a gang. I can blink and be back, age nine, stealing pennies and quarters to get some food for my brother and sister. Eating spaghetti every night month on month. The trailer I was raised in, holes in the floor where blackberry bushes would grow up into the bedrooms.

Now I wear a suit when I like, but I still have the street in me.

The big change came when I found books, and I devoured them while I was in prison. I read books that changed my world. I read every book I could find on wealth and change and possibility. I read every inspirational book I could put my hands on and began to change.

I began to vision board, and I vision board today. Each day I look at my vision board, and I see where I am against it, and move into it.

When I got out of prison, I started my own moving company, but I still wasn't happy. A few years back, I found a new mentor, and a new lifestyle, and everything changed. I learned how to put faith, family and fitness on par with finance. I began a digital marketing agency that now brings in more per month than some executives bring home in a year. When I look at how much I changed I wanted to share how I changed so much so fast. My values changed. My outlook changed.

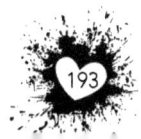

Secret Sauce

The 4 Fs changed me. I use this focus every day...

> Family
> Finance
> Fitness
> Faith

I read that somewhere, I'm not going to take credit for it.

I am not the richest, smartest, or the most talented person in the world.

I shifted out of my grind and chose a new way of life. My wife and I built vision boards and set goals in each of these areas. Every day we look at the goals and we align ourselves with the actions it takes to reach them.

Mindset

I take responsibility for my life now. I think back then, when I was a kid, doing burglaries and robberies, I would look at the rich people and want what they had. I made excuses. I saw myself as a kind of Robin Hood, stealing from the rich (them) to give to the poor (me).

I stopped making excuses. The sign in my office says "F*** Excuses" and I believe that completely.

A lot of us, say and think that we take responsibility only to be accepting this on a surface level.

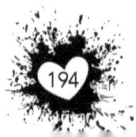

True successful entrepreneurs not only take responsibility/ownership but they constantly put massive action behind finding areas to take responsibility, and change anything and everything that stands in their way to their goals.

Ditch your excuses, take and find ownership to scale and grow! You might need to take some time and find your why.

Finding your WHY sometimes hurts, it's not easy being true with yourself when you have spent your whole life being fake and living on the surface. Most of us don't even know that we are surface living, but if you see that you are, what are you going to do about it?

If you want to be successful in 2019 you're going to have to dig deep to find your WHY....

You're going to have to relive some emotions that you don't like....

You're going to have to cut some people off that you love....

and you're are going to have to start living with focus and discipline.

But the reward outweighs the alternative.

Look for Joshua's new book coming soon.

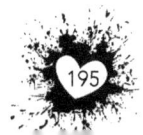

About the Author

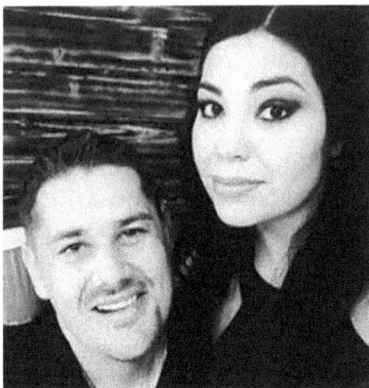

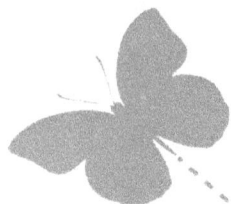

Joshua T. Osborne
www.JoshuaTOsborne.com

THE END

www.ingramcontent.com/pod-product-compliance
Lightning Source LLC
Chambersburg PA
CBHW072001040426
42447CB00009B/1436